As per
NCISM
Competency-Based
BAMS Curriculum
2026

2026 EDITION

PRACTICAL MANUAL OF AGADATANTRA EVAM VIDHI VAIDYAKA

Visha Chikitsa

Agada Dravyas

Observation Records, Medico-Legal Documentation, Toxicology Practical's, Mandatory Educational Visits Report Writing

Toxicology Practicals

Forensic Examination

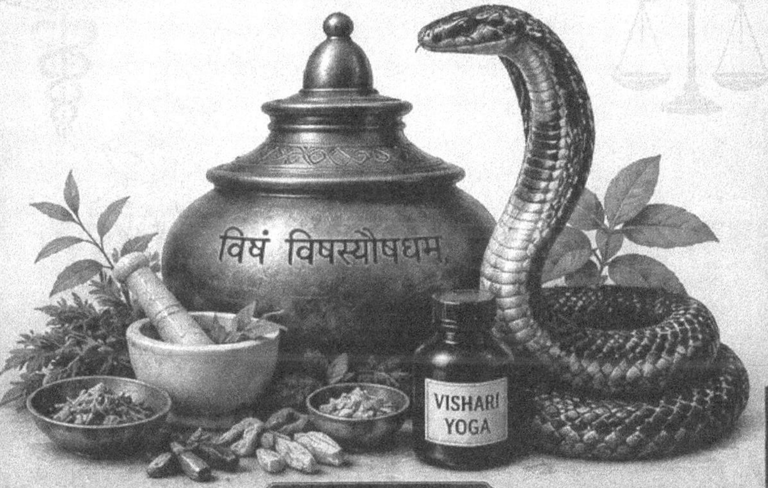

Medico-Legal Documentation

Autopsy & Postmortem

Forensic & Legal Sciences

Court Visit & Report Writing

INCLUDING

- Toxicology Practical Records
- Poison Identification Charts
- Medico-Legal Case Documentation
- Injury & Certificate Drafting
- Autopsy & Court Visit Records
- Educational Visit Reports
- Viva Questions & Competency Assessment
- Observation Record Formats

KNOWLEDGE · PRACTICE · DOCUMENTATION · EXCELLENCE

AUTHOR

Dr. Anil Kumar Y

B.A.M.S., M.D. (Ayu – Agadatantra)
Assistant Professor
Department of Agadatantra Evam Vidhi Vaidyaka
TMAE'S Ayurvedic Medical College,
PG Research Centre & SCS Hospital
Hospet – 583201, Karnataka

Bridging Classical Agadatantra with Modern Toxicology and Medico-Legal Practice

PRACTICAL MANUAL OF AGADATANTRA EVAM VIDHI VAIDYAKA

Observation Records, Medico-Legal Documentation, Toxicology Practical's, Mandatory Educational Visits Report Writing

As per NCISM Competency-Based BAMS Curriculum

2026

AUTHOR

Dr. Anil Kumar Y
B.A.M.S., M.D. (Ayu-Agadatantra)

वैद्यः शास्त्रसम्पन्नो दक्षः शुचिरनन्यधीः

A physician must be Learned, Skilful, Disciplined, and Dedicated.

COPYRIGHT PAGE

PRACTICAL MANUAL OF AGADATANTRA EVAM VIDHI VAIDYAKA

Observation Records, Toxicology Practical's, Medico-Legal Documentation, Educational Visits.

Author:
Dr. Anil Kumar Y
B.A.M.S., M.D. (Ayu) – Agadatantra

First Edition: 2026

ISBN: 9798180205087
Imprint: Visha Vaidya

Published by: Visha Vaidya Publications

Printed in India

For bulk orders, academic adoption, workshops, lectures, or professional correspondence, contact:

Dr. Anil Kumar Y
Email: anilkumar12y@gmail.com
Phone/WhatsApp: +91 8073234223

FOREWORD

It gives me immense pleasure to present this valuable academic work titled "PRACTICAL MANUAL OF AGADATANTRA EVAM VIDHI VAIDYAKA" authored by Dr. Anil Kumar Y, B.A.M.S., M.D. (Ayu - Agadatantra). This book is a sincere and commendable effort aimed at simplifying the vast and clinically important subject of Agadatantra Evam Vidhi Vaidyaka for undergraduate Ayurveda students.

Agadatantra, being one of the essential branches of Ayurveda, deals not only with toxicology and poison management but also with medico-legal aspects that are highly relevant in present-day medical practice. Students often find this subject extensive and challenging. This book has been thoughtfully designed to make learning easier, systematic, examination-oriented, and clinically applicable.

The author has incorporated simplified explanations, mnemonics, diagrams, tables, flowcharts, important examination points, discussions, and conceptual summaries in a student-friendly manner. Such an approach will undoubtedly help students improve their understanding, academic performance, and confidence in the subject.

I appreciate the dedicated efforts of Dr. Anil Kumar Y in preparing this useful "Practical Manual" with a vision to support Ayurveda students and teachers alike. His academic enthusiasm, subject expertise, and commitment towards innovative teaching methods are clearly reflected throughout this work.

I am confident that "PRACTICAL MANUAL OF AGADATANTRA EVAM VIDHI VAIDYAKA " will serve as a beneficial companion for B.A.M.S. students, interns, postgraduate aspirants, and teaching faculty. I congratulate the author for this scholarly contribution and wish him continued success in his academic and literary endeavors.

With Best Wishes,

DR. LEELADHAR D V

PRINCIPAL

K.V.G Ayurveda Medical College & Hospital

Ambate Adka, Kurunjibag,
Sullia DK Dist., Karnataka -
574327 **08257�233208,**
233608

7353756060 / 9449717171

E-mail: principalkvgamc@gmail.com

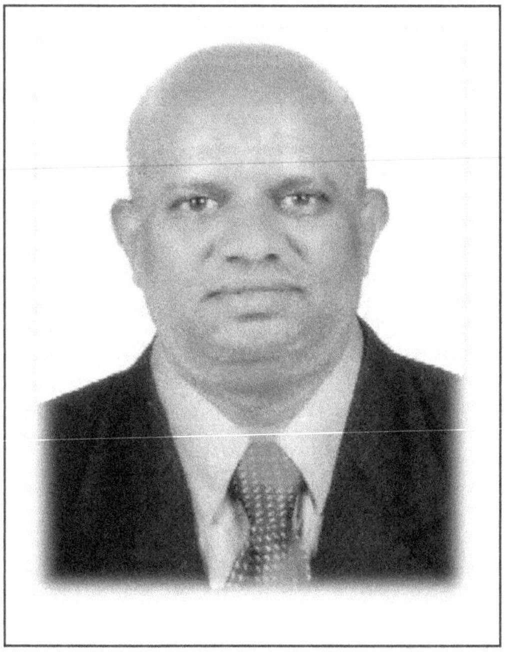

PRACTICAL MANUAL OF AGADATANTRA EVAM VIDHI VAIDYAKA

____________________________________ AYURVEDA MEDICAL

COLLEGE, PLACE_______________________________

PRACTICAL RECORD OBSERVATION BOOK

AGAD TANTRA EVAM VIDHI VAIDYAKA (AyUG-AT)

Student Name: _______________________

BAMS Year: _________________________

Register No.: _______________________

Academic Year: _____________________

Submitted To:
Department of Agadatantra

Signature of Student: _____________

Department of Agadatantra

Signature of Teacher: _____________

Head of Department: _____________

Sl. No.	Practical Topic	Term	Hours
1	Visha Chikitsa (Management of Poisoning)	I	6
2	Vishakta Ahara Pariksha	I	6
3	Dooshivisha, Garavisha, Visha Upadrava	I	20
4	Dermatological Manifestations of Visha	II	20
5	Environmental Toxicology	II	2
6	Jangama Visha	II	10
7	Sthavara Visha	II	6
8	Substance Abuse	III	8
9	Legal Procedures	I	2
10	Vaidya Sadvritta	I	2
11	Personal Identity	I	4
12	Thanatology	II	6
13	Injury	II	6
14	Sexual Offences	III	2
15	Field Visits*	II	30
16	Topics Related to Regional Preference	III	10

Total Practical Hours = 140

Practical Examination Distribution (100 Marks)

- Spotting – 60 Marks
- Practical Records – 10 Marks
- Medical & Medico-legal Certificate Writing – 10 Marks
- Short Case – 10 Marks
- Clinical Applications of Agada Tantra – 10 Marks

Field Visits Include

- Snake parks / serpentariums
- Poison information centres
- Forensic science laboratories
- Toxicology laboratories
- Environmental pollution monitoring centres
- De-addiction centres (where available)

PRACTICAL MANUAL OF AGADATANTRA EVAM VIDHI VAIDYAKA

As Per NCISM II BAMS Curriculum (140 Practical Hours)

The practical record should cover all 16 practical areas prescribed under the NCISM AyUG-AT syllabus.

-- **AYURVEDA MEDICAL COLLEGE**------------------

PRACTICAL RECORD OBSERVATION BOOK

CERTIFICATE

Certified that Mr./Ms. ______________________ has satisfactorily completed the practical work prescribed in **Agad Tantra Evam Vidhi Vaidyaka (AyUG-AT)** during the academic year __________.

Faculty Signature: __________

HOD Signature: __________

Seal

INDEX

PROCEDURE OF GASTRIC LAVAGE ON MANNEQUIN

AIM: To demonstrate the technique of gastric lavage on a mannequin to remove poison or irritant material from the stomach.

INDICATIONS

- Ingestion of poison within 1–2 hours
- Drug overdose
- Unknown poison
- Preparatory to specific antidote

CONTRAINDICATIONS

- Corrosive ingestion (acid/alkali)
- Hydrocarbon ingestion (petrol, kerosene)
- Unconscious patient without airway protection
- Risk of aspiration

EQUIPMENTS REQUIRED

- Stomach tube (wide bore) – Charrière 28–36 (adult)
- Funnel/Fluids
- Kidney tray
- Lubricant (water soluble jelly)
- Tongue depressor
- Towel
- Stethoscope
- Gloves
- Mug with warm water (37–40°C)
- Emesis basin / Bucket

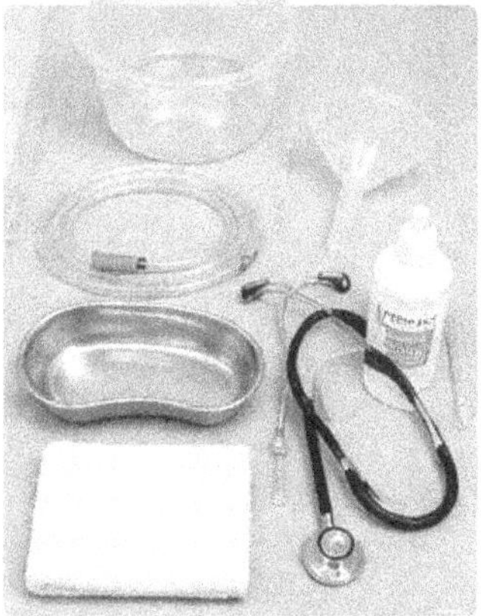

PREPARATION

- Explain the procedure.
- Check all equipments.
- Adjust the mannequin in supine position with head extended.
- Protect clothing with a towel.
- Wear gloves.

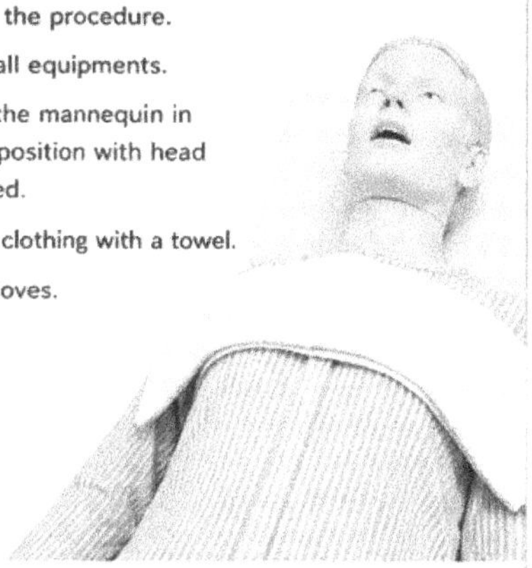

PROCEDURE

1 Measure the required length of the tube. (From tip of nose to ear lobe to xiphisternum in adult.)

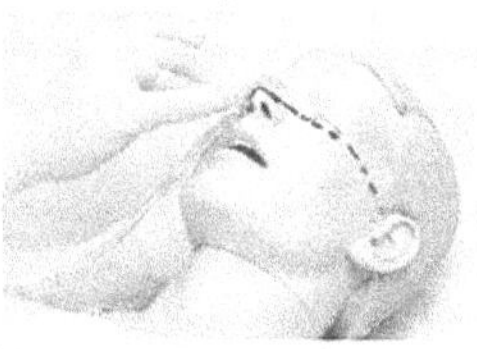

2 Lubricate the stomach tube well.

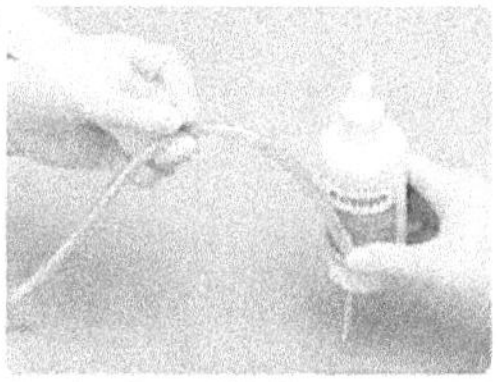

3 Insert the tube gently through the nostril along the floor of the nose.

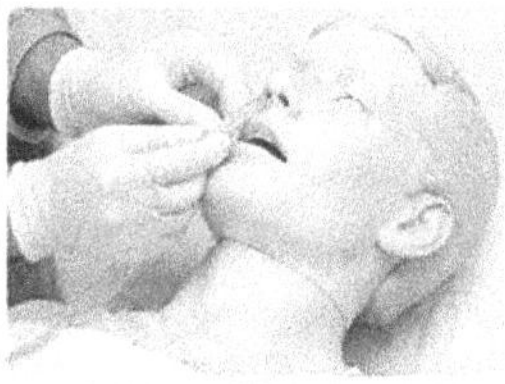

4 Advance the tube slowly up to the measured mark.

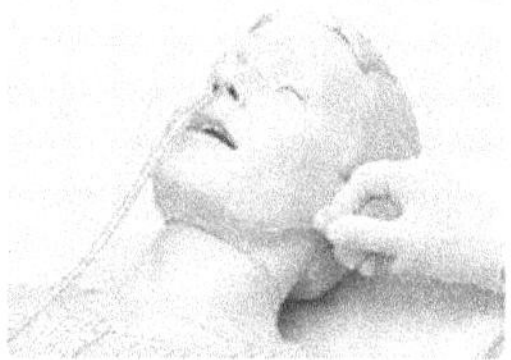

5 Confirm the position of the tube in the stomach by one of the methods:

- Aspirate the gastric contents.
- Inject air and listen over epigastrium (stethoscope test).

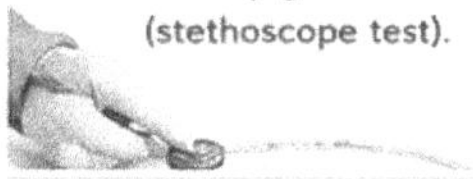

6 Fix the tube in position with adhesive tape.

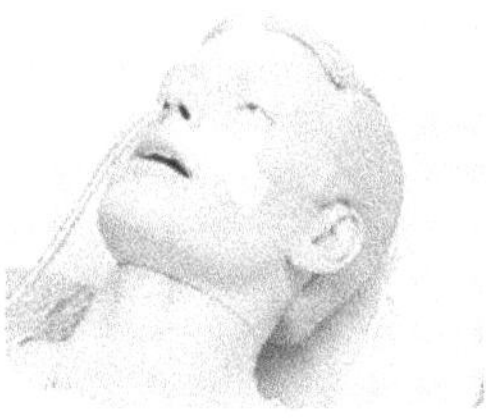

7 Pour warm water (200 – 300 ml) into the funnel.

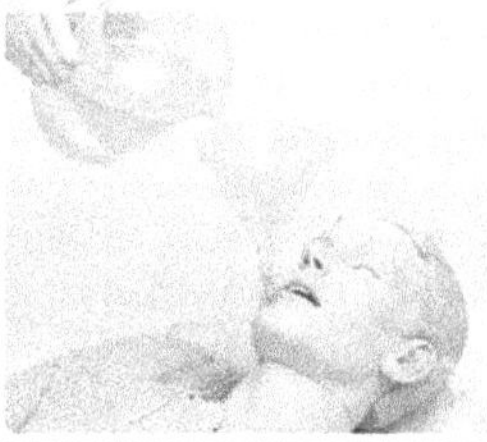

8 Allow the fluid to flow into the stomach by gravity.

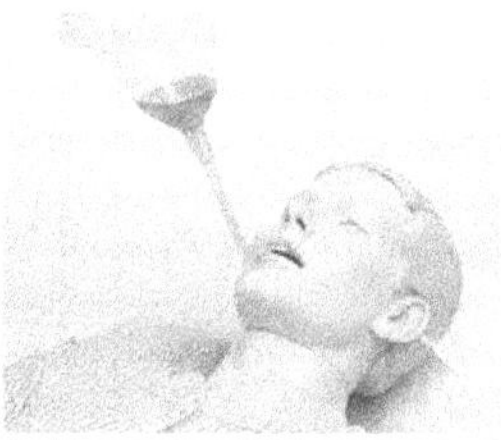

9 Lower the funnel and allow the stomach contents to drain out completely.

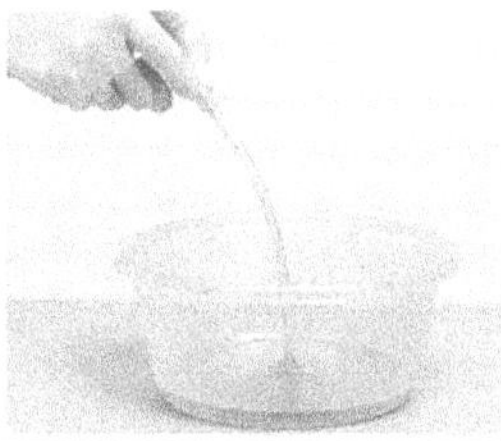

10 Repeat the process until the returning fluid is clear.

Usually 5–10 litres of water may be required in adults.

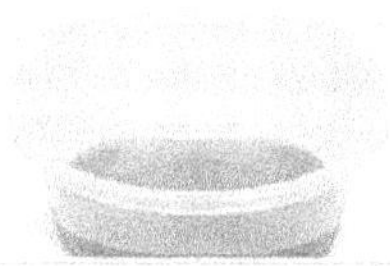

Note: Always monitor the flow. Do not force the tube. Stop the procedure if resistance is felt.

AFTER PROCEDURE

- Remove the tube gently.
- Clean the mannequin.
- Dispose the fluid properly.
- Record the procedure.

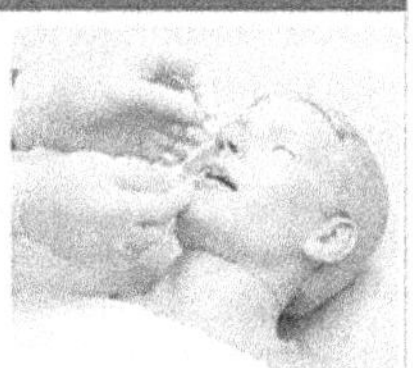

POSSIBLE COMPLICATIONS

- Aspiration of vomitus
- Injury to nose, pharynx or oesophagus
- Laryngospasm
- Fluid and electrolyte imbalance
- Hypothermia
- Perforation (rare)

KEY POINTS

- Gastric lavage is most effective within 1–2 hours of poisoning.
- Use wide bore tube for better flow.
- Use warm water (not hot or cold).
- Maintain airway protection in unconscious patient.
- Perform the procedure gently and patiently.

CONCLUSION

Gastric lavage is an important decontamination procedure in poisoning cases when performed early and correctly.

PRECAUTIONS

- Do not perform in corrosive or hydrocarbon ingestion.
- Ensure correct placement of the tube before starting lavage.
- Maintain warmth and observe for any complications.

PRACTICAL NO. 1

1.1 VISHA CHIKITSA

Date:

Practical Title: Procedure of Gastric Lavage on mannequin.

Aim:

Materials Required

Mnemonic: "WASH STOMACH"

W – Wear protective equipment
A – Assess airway, breathing, circulation (ABC)
S – Select appropriate tube (orogastric tube)
H – Head lowered in left lateral position

S – Stomach contents aspirated first
T – Test tube position
O – Open lavage with warm normal saline/water
M – Measure instilled fluid
A – Aspirate back the fluid
C – Continue till clear return
H – Handle samples for toxicological analysis

Procedure:

Observations:

Results:

Discussion:

C – Corrosive poisoning (strong acids/alkalis)
A – Airway unprotected/unconscious without intubation
U – Uncontrolled seizures
S – Sharp objects ingested
T – Threat of perforation/bleeding
I – Ingestion of hydrocarbons (kerosene, petrol) with aspiration risk
C – Compromised respiratory status

Teacher Signature

PROCEDURE OF CARDIOPULMONARY RESUSCITATION (CPR) ON MANNEQUIN

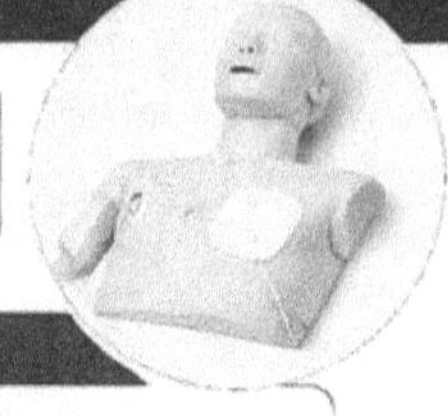

AIM: To demonstrate the technique of Cardiopulmonary Resuscitation (CPR) on a mannequin to maintain circulation and oxygenation in a victim of cardiac arrest.

INDICATIONS

- Cardiac arrest
- Unresponsiveness
- No normal breathing
- No pulse

OBJECTIVES

- To maintain airway patency
- To maintain circulation
- To maintain oxygenation until advanced care arrives

INITIAL ASSESSMENT

A ASSESS SAFETY

Ensure the area is safe for rescuer and victim.

B CHECK RESPONSE

Tap the mannequin and shout. "No response".

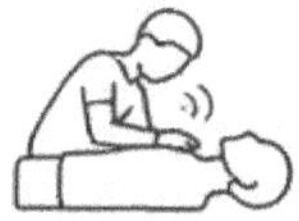

C CHECK BREATHING

Open airway, look, listen and feel for breathing for 10 seconds. No normal breathing.

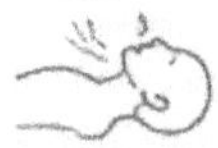

D ACTIVATE EMERGENCY RESPONSE

Call for help/ Activate EMS and get AED if available.

CPR PROCEDURE (Adult)

1 POSITION THE MANNEQUIN

Place the mannequin on a firm, flat surface.

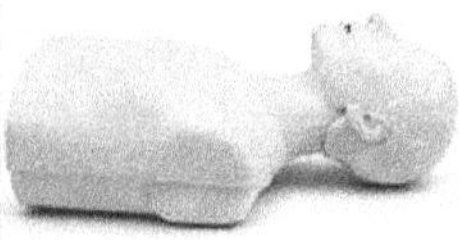

2 OPEN THE AIRWAY

Tilt the head back slightly and lift the chin.

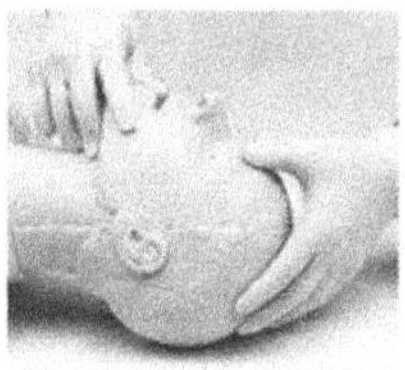

3 CHECK BREATHING AGAIN

Look, listen and feel for breathing for 10 seconds.

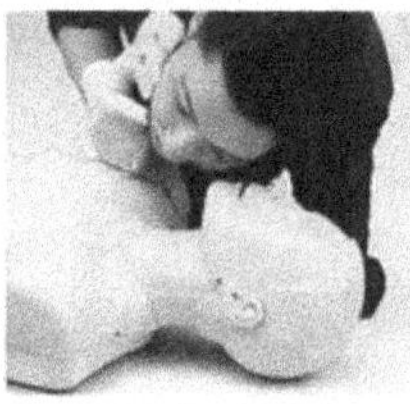

4 CHEST COMPRESSIONS

Place heel of one hand on the center of chest (lower half of sternum), other hand on top.

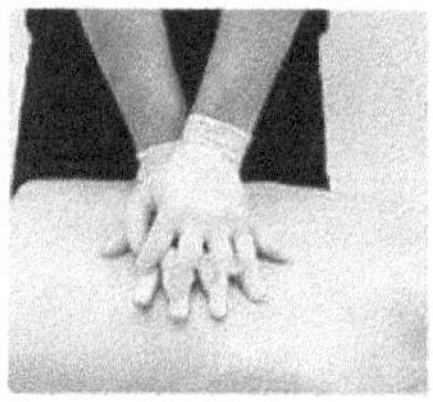

5 PERFORM COMPRESSIONS

Push hard and fast.
- Rate: 100–120/min
- Depth: 5–6 cm
- Allow full recoil

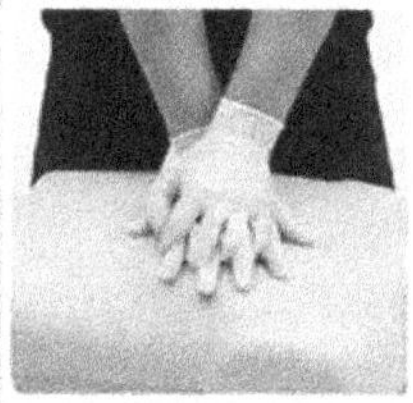

6 GIVE VENTILATIONS

After 30 compressions, open airway and give 2 rescue breaths. (Each breath 1 sec)

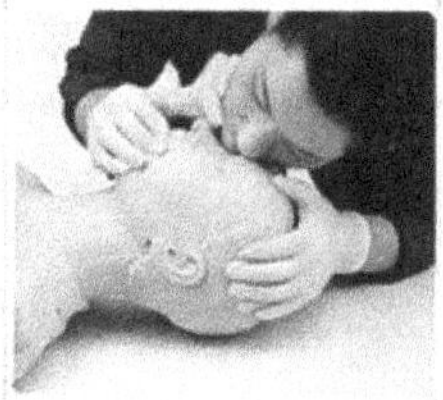

CYCLE: 30 COMPRESSIONS : 2 BREATHS **Continue cycles without interruption.**

RESCUE BREATHS – TECHNIQUE

- Open the airway (Head tilt–chin lift).
- Pinch the nose.
- Take a normal breath, seal your lips around the mouth of mannequin.
- Blow steadily for about 1 second and watch the chest rise.
- Remove your mouth and allow chest to fall.
- Give second breath.

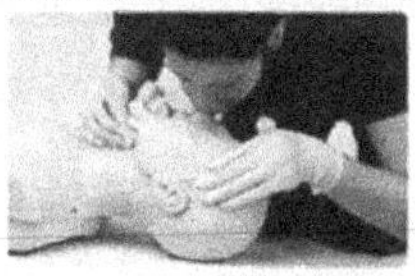

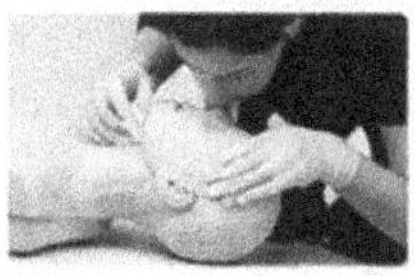

USE OF AED (If Available)

1. Switch on the AED.
2. Attach the pads to the mannequin as per diagram.
3. Ensure no one is touching the mannequin.
4. Allow AED to analyze the rhythm.
5. If shock advised – deliver shock.
6. Immediately resume CPR for 2 minutes (30:2 ratio) and follow AED prompts.

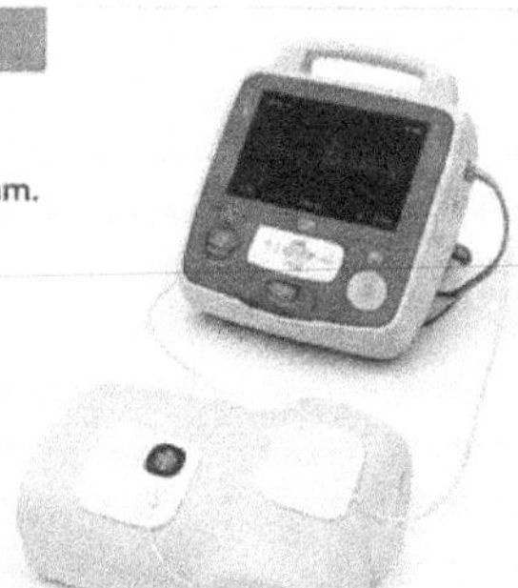

KEY POINTS

- Ensure correct hand position and depth of compression.
- Maintain compression rate 100–120/min.
- Minimize interruptions in compressions.
- Effective CPR is a balance of chest compressions and ventilations.

COMPRESSION-VENTILATION RATIO

Adult	Child / Infant
30 : 2	30 : 2
One Rescuer	Two Rescuers

SIGNS OF EFFECTIVE CPR

- Chest rises with every breath.
- Palpable pulse (if checked).
- Improved color of mannequin.

PRECAUTIONS

- Ensure the surface is firm and flat.
- Do not over-ventilate.
- Avoid excessive interruption.
- Follow universal precautions.

CONCLUSION

CPR is a life-saving procedure that helps maintain circulation and oxygenation during cardiac arrest until advanced medical care is provided.

1.2 VISHA CHIKITSA

Date:

Practical Title: Procedure of Cardiopulmonary Resuscitation (CPR) On Mannequin.

Aim:

Materials Required

Procedure:

Reversible Causes of Cardiac Arrest

Mnemonic: 5 H's and 5 T's

5 H's

- **Hypoxia**
- **Hypovolemia**
- **Hydrogen ion (Acidosis)**
- **Hypo/Hyperkalemia**
- **Hypothermia**

5 T's

- **Tension Pneumothorax**
- **Tamponade (Cardiac)**
- **Toxins**
- **Thrombosis (Coronary)**
- **Thrombosis (Pulmonary)**

Observations:

Results:

Discussion:

DRS CAB

D

Danger – Ensure scene safety

R

Response – Check responsiveness

S

Send for help / Activate emergency response

C

Chest compressions

A

Airway

B

Breathing

Mnemonic:
☞ **"Don't Rush, Send Care And Breaths"**

Teacher Signature

1.3 VISHA CHIKITSA

Date:

Practical Title: **Procedures for Removal of Absorbed poison.**

Aim:

Materials Required

Procedure:

Observations:

Results:

Discussion:

Teacher Signature

PROCEDURES FOR REMOVAL OF ABSORBED POISON

DEFINITION: Removal of absorbed poison refers to therapeutic measures adopted to eliminate or reduce poison already absorbed into systemic circulation.

METHODS FOR REMOVAL OF ABSORBED POISON

1. FORCED DIURESIS

PRINCIPLE:
Enhances urinary excretion of poison by increasing urine output.

PROCEDURE:
- Administer intravenous fluids.
- Use diuretics such as Furosemide.
- Monitor urine output and electrolytes.

INDICATIONS:
- Salicylates
- Barbiturates
- Phenobarbital

CONTRAINDICATIONS:
- Renal failure
- Pulmonary edema
- Cardiac failure

2. URINARY ALKALINIZATION

PRINCIPLE:
Alkalinization of urine increases excretion of acidic poisons.

PROCEDURE:
- Administer Sodium bicarbonate intravenously.
- Maintain urine pH around 7.5 – 8.

INDICATIONS:
- Salicylate poisoning
- Phenobarbital poisoning

NOTE:
Monitor urine pH frequently.
Maintain adequate hydration.

3. URINARY ACIDIFICATION

PRINCIPLE:
Acidification enhances elimination of alkaline drugs.

PROCEDURE:
- Administer ammonium chloride or ascorbic acid carefully.

INDICATIONS:
- Rarely used today
- Amphetamine poisoning

NOTE:
Usually avoided due to complications like acidosis and tissue irritation.

4. HEMODIALYSIS

PRINCIPLE:
Removes poison directly from blood through dialysis membrane.

PROCEDURE:
- Blood is passed through dialysis machine.
- Poison diffuses across semipermeable membrane.

INDICATIONS:
- Methanol poisoning
- Ethylene glycol poisoning
- Severe salicylate poisoning
- Lithium poisoning
- Renal failure associated poisoning

ADVANTAGES:
- Rapid toxin removal
- Corrects electrolyte imbalance
- Useful in severe poisonings

5. HEMOPERFUSION

PRINCIPLE:
Blood passes through adsorbent material such as activated charcoal or resin.

PROCEDURE:
- Blood is circulated through a cartridge containing adsorbent.
- Toxin is adsorbed and removed.

INDICATIONS:
- Theophylline poisoning
- Carbamazepine poisoning
- Barbiturate poisoning
- Paraquat poisoning

NOTE:
Less effective than hemodialysis but useful for protein-bound toxins.

6. EXCHANGE TRANSFUSION

PRINCIPLE:
Poisoned blood is removed and replaced with fresh blood.

PROCEDURE:
- Remove small volume of patient's blood.
- Replace with equal volume of donor blood.
- Repeat until clinical improvement.

INDICATIONS:
- Severe neonatal poisoning
- Certain drug toxicities (e.g., theophylline)
- Hemolytic poisonings

7. CHELATION THERAPY

PRINCIPLE:
Chelating agents bind heavy metals and enhance their excretion.

POISON	CHELATING AGENT	ROUTE
Lead	Calcium EDTA	IV
Arsenic	BAL (Dimercaprol)	IM / IV
Mercury	BAL (Dimercaprol)	IM / IV
Copper	Penicillamine	Oral
Iron	Deferoxamine	IV
Zinc	Penicillamine / Ca EDTA	Oral / IV

8. SPECIFIC ANTIDOTAL THERAPY

PRINCIPLE:
Specific antidotes neutralize or counteract the effect of poison.

POISON	ANTIDOTE
Opioids	Naloxone
Organophosphorus compounds	Atropine + Pralidoxime
Methanol	Ethanol / Fomepizole
Cyanide	Sodium nitrite + Sodium thiosulfate
Benzodiazepines	Flumazenil
Warfarin	Vitamin K + FFP
Paracetamol	N-Acetylcysteine
Digoxin	Digoxin Fab fragments

GENERAL PRECAUTIONS

1. Maintain airway, breathing, and circulation.
2. Monitor vitals continuously.
3. Correct fluid and electrolyte imbalance.
4. Avoid delay in antidotal therapy.
5. Identify the poison if possible.
6. Provide supportive care.

IMPORTANT POINTS

- Choice of method depends on type of poison, time of exposure, and patient's condition.
- Early treatment improves outcome.
- These procedures should be carried out in hospital under expert supervision.

CONCLUSION

Removal of absorbed poison is an important aspect of toxicological emergency management aimed at enhancing elimination, reducing toxicity, and preventing complications.

PRACTICAL NO. 2

2.1 VISHAKTA AHARA PARIKSHA

Experiment

1. Detection of Urea in Milk

Aim:

Principle:

Materials:

Procedure:

Observation:

Result:

Teacher Signature

DETECTION OF UREA IN MILK AS PER FSSAI GUIDELINES

Urea is sometimes illegally added to milk to increase the apparent total solids and SNF.
FSSAI has prescribed the Diacetyl Monoxime (DMO) test for the detection of urea in milk.

FSSAI
FOOD SAFETY AND STANDARDS AUTHORITY OF INDIA

(Ref: FSSAI Manual of Methods of Analysis of Foods, 1st Edition, 2015) (Method No. 7.5)

PRINCIPLE

Urea present in milk reacts with Diacetyl Monoxime in acidic medium in the presence of ferric ions to produce a pink to reddish colour.

REQUIREMENTS

- Milk sample
- Diacetyl Monoxime (DMO) solution (1% in ethanol)
- Concentrated Hydrochloric acid (HCl)
- Ferric Chloride solution (10%)
- Test tubes, Pipettes

PROCEDURE

1. Take 5 ml of milk sample in a test tube.
2. Add 1 ml of Diacetyl Monoxime (DMO) solution (1%).
3. Add 1 ml of concentrated HCl slowly along the side of the test tube.
4. Add 1 ml of Ferric Chloride solution (10%).
5. Mix gently using a glass rod.
6. Observe the colour change within 2–3 minutes.

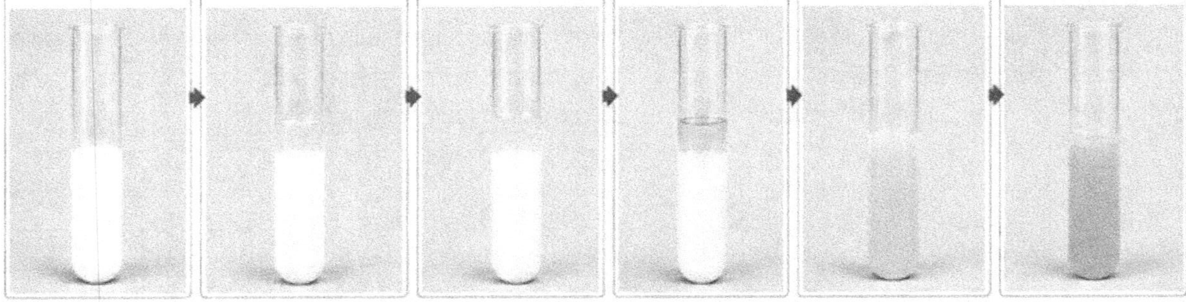

OBSERVATION AND INFERENCE

Observation	Inference
Pink to reddish colour develops in the upper layer	Urea is PRESENT (Milk is adulterated)
No pink colour / No change (Yellowish layer remains)	Urea is ABSENT (Milk is pure)

CHEMICAL REACTION

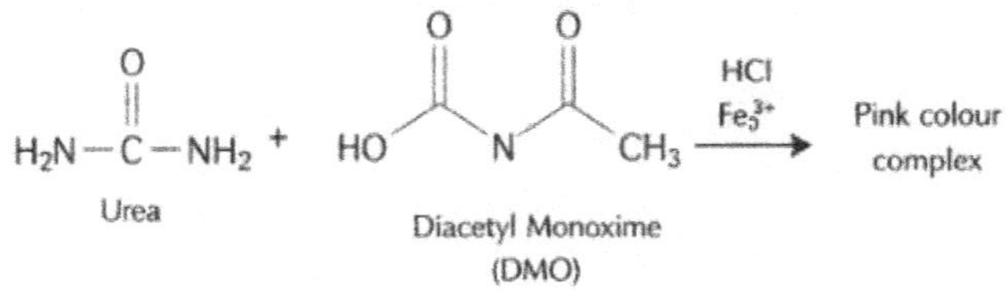

Urea + DMO (in acidic medium with ferric ions) → Pink coloured complex

NOTE

- Urea is not permitted in milk as per FSSAI standards.
- Presence of urea indicates adulteration and the milk is unsafe for consumption.
- This is a qualitative test. For confirmation, instrumental methods like HPLC / LC-MS / Enzymatic methods may be used.

PRECAUTIONS

- Use fresh DMO solution.
- Add concentrated HCl carefully along the side of the test tube.
- Do not shake vigorously; mix gently.
- Use clean and dry glassware.

DISPOSAL OF WASTES

- Acidic wastes should be neutralized before disposal.
- Follow laboratory safety and environmental guidelines.

REFERENCE (As per FSSAI Guidelines)

FSSAI Manual of Methods of Analysis of Foods – Food Safety and Standards Authority of India 1st Edition, 2015, Method No. 7.5

CONCLUSION: The above test helps in detecting urea in milk as per FSSAI guidelines and ensures food safety and consumer protection.

PRACTICAL NO. 2

2.1 VISHAKTA AHARA PARIKSHA

Experiment

2. Detection of Boric Acid in Milk

Aim:

Principle:

Materials:

Procedure:

Observation:

Result:

Teacher Signature

DETECTION OF BORIC ACID IN MILK AS PER FSSAI GUIDELINES

Boric acid is sometimes illegally added to milk to prevent microbial growth and increase shelf life. FSSAI has prescribed the Curcumin (Turmeric) paper test for the detection of boric acid in milk.

FOOD SAFETY AND STANDARDS AUTHORITY OF INDIA

(Ref: FSSAI Manual of Methods of Analysis of Foods, 1st Edition, 2015) (Method No. 7.7)

PRINCIPLE

Boric acid present in milk reacts with curcumin in turmeric paper in the presence of dehydrating agent (Quandong resin / hydrochloric acid) to give a red colour.

REQUIREMENTS

- Milk sample
- Curcumin (turmeric) paper strips
- Conc. Hydrochloric acid (HCl) or sulfuric acid
- Quandong resin solution (10%)
- Test tubes, Pipettes, Glass rod

PROCEDURE

1 Take 5 ml of milk sample in a test tube.

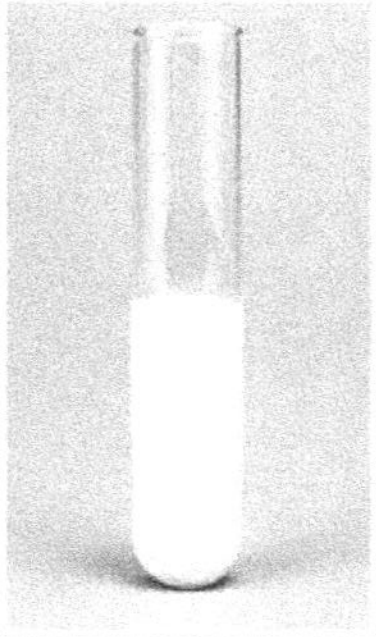

2 Add 1 ml of Quandong resin solution (10%).

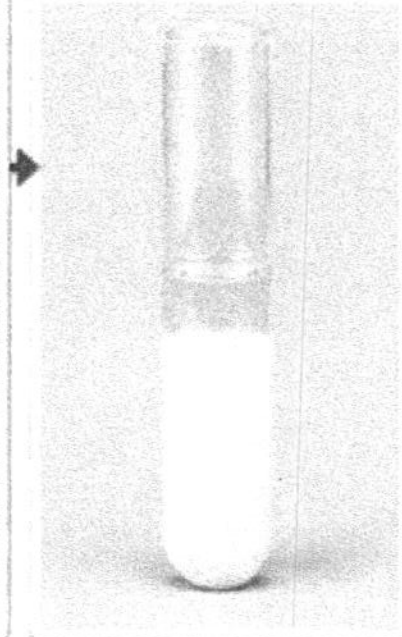

3 Add 1 ml of concentrated HCl.

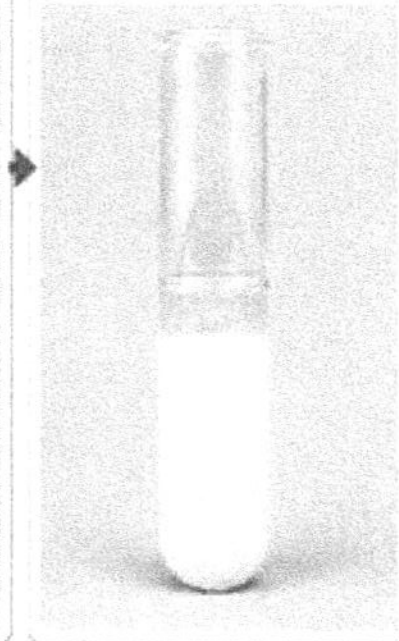

4 Mix well and allow to stand for 1–2 minutes.

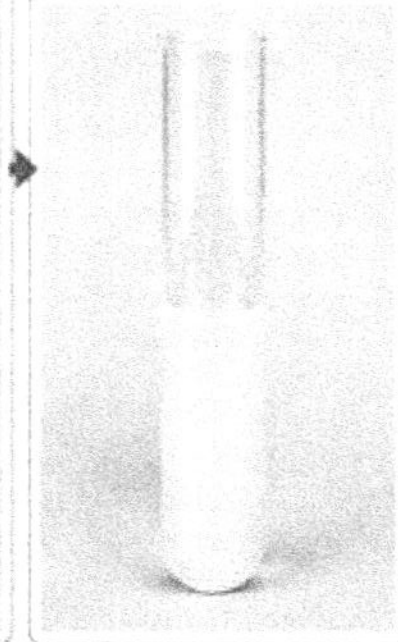

5 Dip the curcumin (turmeric) paper strip in the solution.

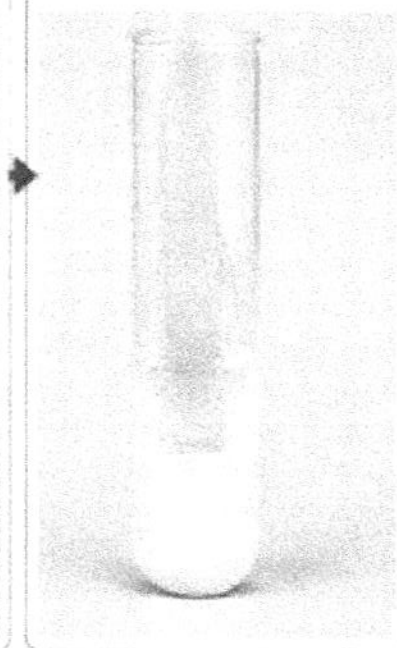

6 Observe the colour change after 2 minutes.

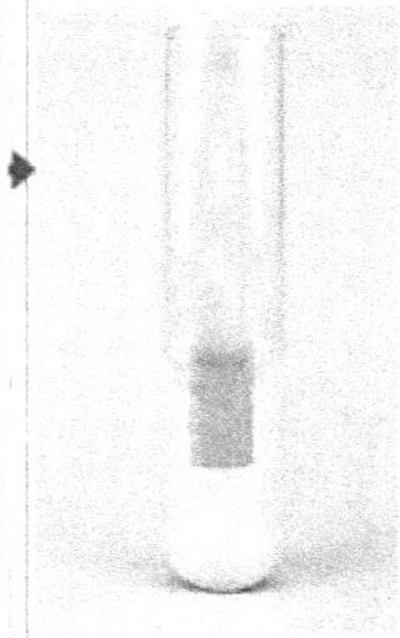

OBSERVATION AND INFERENCE

Observation	Inference
Curcumin paper turns red / reddish-brown	Boric acid is PRESENT (Milk is adulterated)
No change in colour (yellow remains)	Boric acid is ABSENT (Milk is pure)

CHEMICAL REACTION

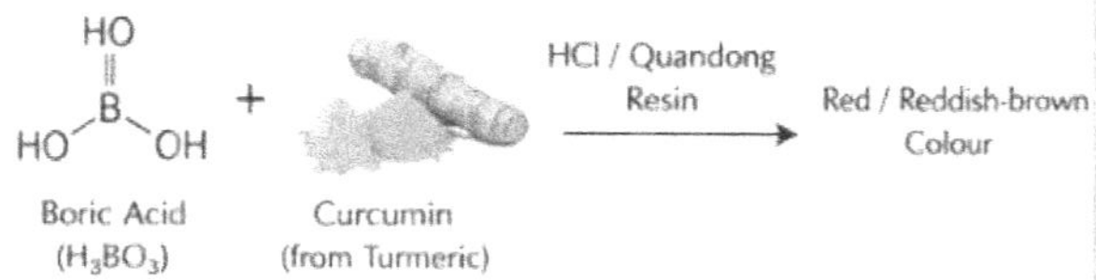

Boric acid + Curcumin (in acidic medium) ⟶ Red colour complex

NOTE

- Boric acid is not permitted in milk as per FSSAI standards.
- Presence of boric acid indicates adulteration and the milk is unsafe for consumption.
- This is a qualitative test. For confirmation, instrumental methods like HPLC / ICP-MS may be used.

PRECAUTIONS

- Use freshly prepared curcumin paper.
- Use clean and dry test tubes.
- Handle acids and resin carefully.
- Do not touch the reactive end of the paper strip.

DISPOSAL OF WASTES

- Acidic wastes should be neutralized before disposal.
- Follow laboratory safety and environmental guidelines.

REFERENCE (As per FSSAI Guidelines)

FSSAI Manual of Methods of Analysis of Foods – Food Safety and Standards Authority of India 1st Edition, 2015, Method No. 7.7

CONCLUSION: The above test helps in detecting boric acid in milk as per FSSAI guidelines and ensures food safety and consumer protection.

PRACTICAL NO. 2

2.1 VISHAKTA AHARA PARIKSHA

Experiment

3. Detection of Artificial Colour in Turmeric

Aim:

Principle:

Materials:

Procedure:

Observation:

Result:

Teacher Signature

DETECTION OF ARTIFICIAL COLOUR IN TURMERIC AS PER FSSAI GUIDELINES

Turmeric is often coloured artificially with non-permitted colours such as Metanil Yellow.
FSSAI has prescribed method for the detection of these artificial colours in turmeric powder.

FOOD SAFETY AND STANDARDS AUTHORITY OF INDIA

(Ref: FSSAI Manual of Methods of Analysis of Foods, 1st Edition, 2015) (Method No. 6.5)

PRINCIPLE

Artificial colours, if present in turmeric, are extracted with suitable solvent and identified by the characteristic colour in acid and alkali media.

REQUIREMENTS

- Turmeric powder
- Acetone
- Concentrated Hydrochloric acid (HCl)
- 10% Sodium Hydroxide (NaOH) solution
- Test tubes, Beaker, Filter paper, Glass rod, Pipettes

PROCEDURE

1. Take 5 g of turmeric powder in a beaker.
2. Add 25 ml of acetone and stir well.
3. Filter the extract using filter paper.
4. Take 5 ml of the filtrate in a test tube.
5. Add 2–3 drops of concentrated HCl.
6. Then add 2–3 drops of 10% NaOH solution.

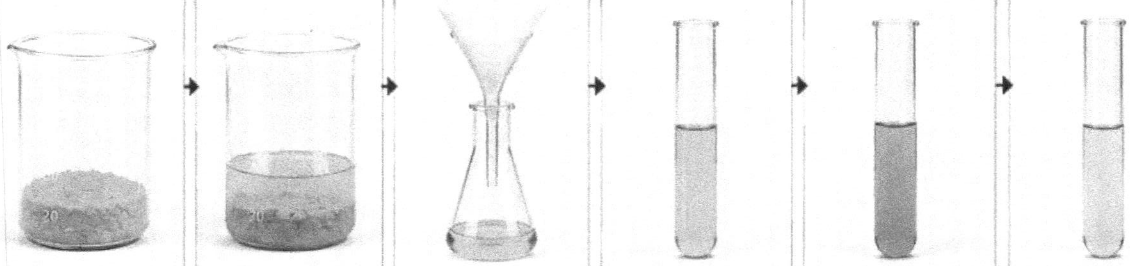

OBSERVATION AND INFERENCE

Observation in Acid (HCl)	Observation in Alkali (NaOH)	Inference
Pink to red	Yellow	Presence of artificial colour (e.g. Metanil Yellow)
No change (remains yellow)	No change (remains yellow)	No artificial colour detected (Sample is pure)
Red	Yellow	Presence of artificial colour (other than Metanil Yellow)

CONFIRMATION OF COLOURS (Guide)

Artificial Colour	In Acid (HCl)	In Alkali (NaOH)
Metanil Yellow	Pink to Red	Yellow
Sunset Yellow FCF	Red	Yellow
Tartrazine	Orange	Yellow
Sudan Red	Red	Yellow

NOTE

- Only permitted colours as per FSSAI standards should be used in foods.
- Presence of non-permitted artificial colour indicates adulteration.
- This method is qualitative. For confirmation, further analysis by TLC / HPLC may be done.
- Ensure proper safety while handling acids, alkalis and organic solvents.

PRECAUTIONS

- Use pure and dry acetone.
- Do not boil the sample.
- Handle concentrated acids and alkalis carefully.
- Use clean and dry glassware.

DISPOSAL OF WASTES

- Acidic and alkaline wastes should be neutralized before disposal.
- Follow laboratory safety and environmental guidelines.

REFERENCE

FSSAI Manual of Methods of Analysis of Foods – Food Safety and Standards Authority of India 1st Edition, 2015, Method No. 6.5

CONCLUSION: The above test helps in detecting artificial colours in turmeric as per FSSAI guidelines and ensures food safety and consumer protection.

PRACTICAL NO. 2

2.2 VISHAKTA AHARA PARIKSHA

Experiment

4. Detection of Artificial Colour in Pulses

Aim:

Principle:

Materials:

Procedure:

Observation:

Result:

Teacher Signature

DETECTION OF ARTIFICIAL COLOUR IN PULSES AS PER FSSAI GUIDELINES

Some pulses are artificially coloured using non-permitted dyes such as Sudan Red, Metanil Yellow, Rhodamine B etc. FSSAI has prescribed methods for the detection of these artificial colours in food samples.

FOOD SAFETY AND STANDARDS AUTHORITY OF INDIA
(Ref: FSSAI Manual of Methods of Analysis of Foods, 1st Edition, 2015). (Method No. 6.5)

PRINCIPLE

Artificial colours, if present in pulses, are extracted using suitable solvent and identified by the characteristic colour in acid and alkali media.

REQUIREMENTS

- Pulse sample (e.g., Tur dal / Masoor dal)
- Acetone
- Concentrated Hydrochloric acid (HCl)
- 10% Sodium Hydroxide (NaOH) solution
- Test tubes, Beaker, Filter paper, Glass rod, Pipettes

PROCEDURE

1. Take 10 g of pulse sample in a beaker.
2. Add 50 ml of acetone.
3. Boil for 2–3 minutes and allow it to cool. Filter the extract.
4. Take 5 ml of the filtrate in a test tube.
5. Add 2–3 drops of concentrated HCl.

Then add 2–3 drops of 10% NaOH solution.

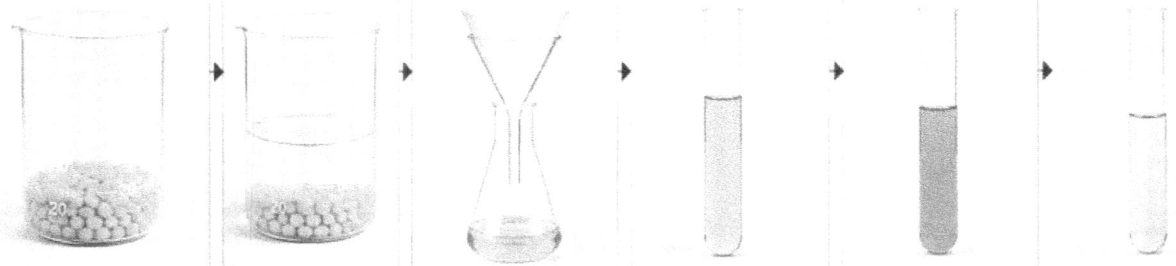

OBSERVATION AND INFERENCE

Observation in HCl (Acidic medium)	Observation in NaOH (Alkaline medium)	Inference (Artificial Colour)
Pink to red	Yellow	Rhodamine B
Red	Yellow	Sudan Red
Yellow	Colourless	Metanil Yellow
No colour change	No colour change	No artificial colour detected

CONFIRMATION OF COLOURS

Artificial Colour	In Acid (HCl)	In Alkali (NaOH)
Rhodamine B	Pink to Red	Yellow
Sudan Red	Red	Yellow
Metanil Yellow	Yellow	Colourless

NOTE

- Only permitted colours as per FSSAI standards should be used in foods.
- Presence of non-permitted artificial colour indicates adulteration.
- This method is qualitative. For confirmation, further analysis by TLC / HPLC may be done.
- Ensure proper safety while handling acids, alkalis and organic solvents.

PRECAUTIONS

- Use pure and dry acetone.
- Do not boil for long duration.
- Handle concentrated acids and alkalis carefully.
- Use glassware free from contamination.

DISPOSAL OF WASTES

- Acidic and alkaline wastes should be neutralized before disposal.
- Follow laboratory safety and environmental guidelines.

REFERENCE (As per FSSAI Guidelines)

FSSAI Manual of Methods of Analysis of Foods – Food Safety and Standards Authority of India 1st Edition, 2015, Method No. 6.5

CONCLUSION: The above test helps in detecting artificial colours in pulses as per FSSAI guidelines and ensures food safety and consumer protection.

PRACTICAL NO. 2

2.2 VISHAKTA AHARA PARIKSHA

Experiment

5. Detection of Argemone Oil in Mustard Oil

Aim:

Principle:

Materials:

Procedure:

Observation:

Result:

Teacher Signature

5. Detection of Argemone Oil in Mustard Oil

DETECTION OF ARGEMONE OIL IN MUSTARD OIL AS PER FSSAI GUIDELINES

Argemone oil is unsafe for human consumption. FSSAI has laid down the method for its detection in edible oils. The method is based on the reaction of sanguinarine (a toxic alkaloid present in Argemone oil) with alcoholic picric acid to give a pink to blood red colour.

fssai

FOOD SAFETY AND STANDARDS AUTHORITY OF INDIA

(Ref: FSSAI Manual of Methods of Analysis of Foods, Oil & Oil Products)

PRINCIPLE

Sanguinarine present in Argemone oil reacts with picric acid in alkaline medium to produce a pink to red colour in the lower layer.

REQUIREMENTS

- Mustard oil sample
- Concentrated Nitric acid (HNO_3)
- Alcoholic Picric acid solution
- Ammonia solution (25%)
- Distilled water
- Test tubes, Pipettes, Separator funnel

PROCEDURE

1	2	3	4	5	6
Take 5 ml of the oil sample in a test tube.	Add 2 ml of concentrated Nitric acid.	Shake well and allow it to stand for 2 minutes.	Add 2 ml of Alcoholic Picric acid solution.	Add 1 ml of Ammonia solution (25%).	Shake gently and allow the layers to separate.

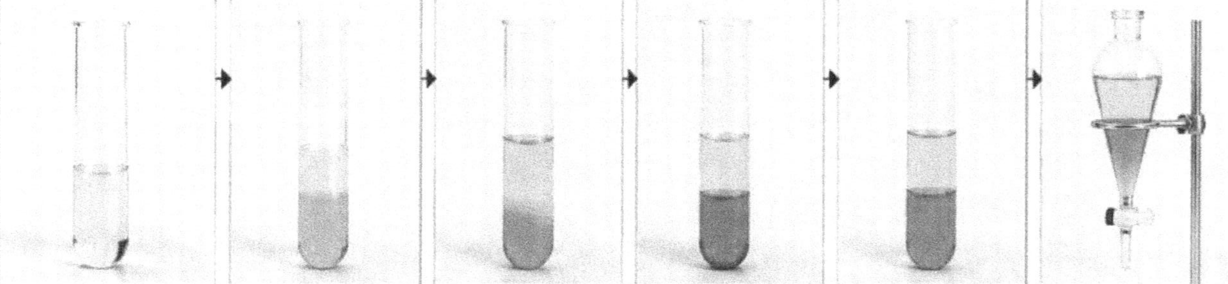

5 ml oil	2 ml HNO_3	Mix and stand	2 ml Picric acid	1 ml NH_3 solution	Allow to separate

OBSERVATION / INFERENCE

OBSERVATION	INFERENCE
Pink to blood red colour in the lower layer	Argemone oil PRESENT (Unsafe for consumption)
No pink or red colour (lower layer remains yellow)	Argemone oil ABSENT (Sample is safe)
Faint pink colour	Argemone oil may be present in low concentration

CHEMICAL REACTION

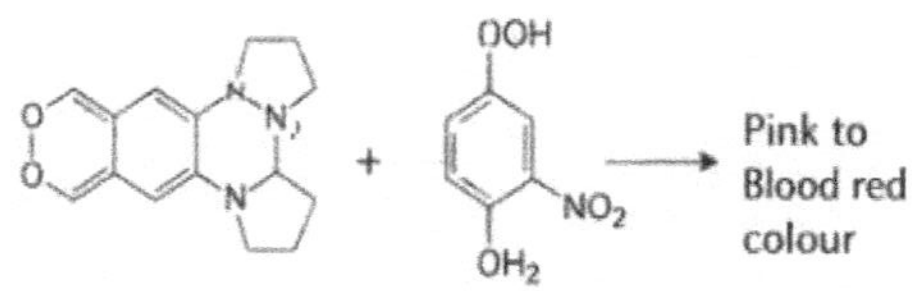

Sanguinarine (from Argemone oil) + Picric acid (Alkaline medium)

NOTE

- Presence of Argemone oil even in small quantity is hazardous.
- FSSAI notifies Argemone oil as a prohibited substance in edible oils.
- This method is qualitative. For confirmation, GC–MS or HPLC can be used.

PRECAUTIONS

- Handle concentrated Nitric acid and Ammonia solution carefully.
- Use clean and dry glassware.
- Do not shake vigorously after adding Ammonia; shake gently.

DISPOSAL OF REAGENTS

- Acidic and alkaline wastes should be neutralized before disposal.
- Follow laboratory safety and environmental guidelines.

REFERENCE (As per FSSAI Guidelines)

FSSAI Manual of Methods of Analysis of Foods – Oil & Oil Products, 1st Edition, 2015. (Method No. 11.7)

PRACTICAL NO. 2

2.2 VISHAKTA AHARA PARIKSHA

Experiment

6. Detection of Adulteration in Honey

Aim:

Principle:

Materials:

Procedure:

Observation:

Result:

Teacher Signature

DETECTION OF ADULTERATION IN HONEY

AIM – To detect the adulteration of honey.

PRINCIPLE – Pure honey does not give characteristic reactions of cane sugar (sucrose) and starch.

REQUIREMENTS – Honey sample, Distilled water, Fehling's solution A & B, Test tube, Dropper, Beaker, Iodine solution.

TESTS AND PROCEDURE

1. FEHLING'S TEST (For added sugar)

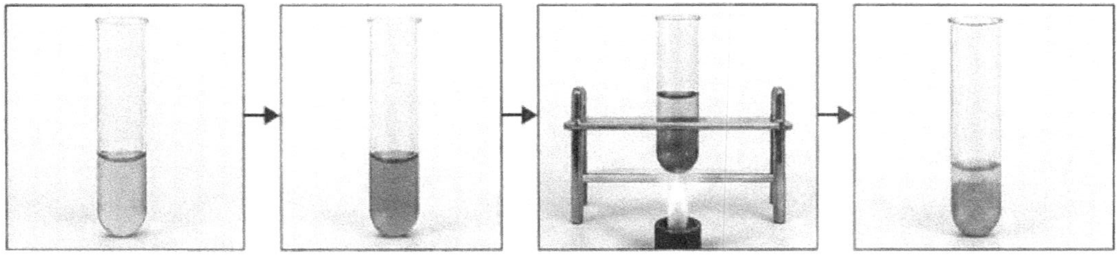

Take 5 ml of honey solution in a test tube. → Add equal volumes of Fehling's A & B. → Boil the mixture for 2–3 minutes. → Formation of brick red precipitate indicates presence of added sugar.

2. IODINE TEST (For added starch)

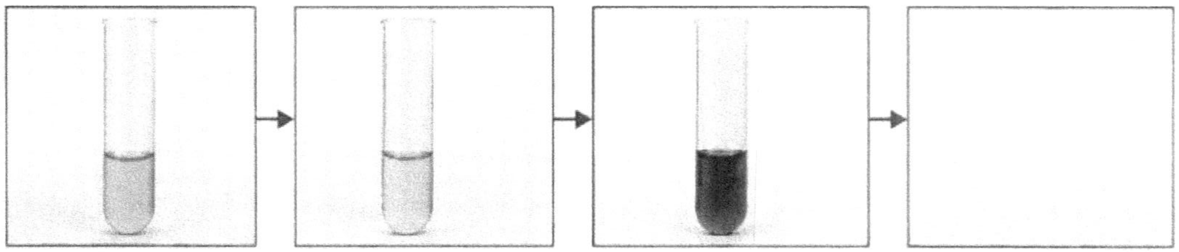

Take 5 ml of honey solution in a test tube. → Add 2–3 drops of iodine solution. → Mix well. → Blue or blue-black colour indicates presence of starch.

OBSERVATION AND INFERENCE

Observation	Inference
Brick red precipitate obtained.	Honey is adulterated with sugar (sucrose/ invert sugar).
No precipitate, solution remains blue.	Honey is pure (no added sugar).

Observation	Inference
Blue / blue-black colour appears.	Honey is adulterated with starch.
No change in colour (yellow-brown).	Honey is pure (no added starch).

CONCLUSION – The above tests help in detecting common adulterants in honey such as added sugar and starch.

PRACTICAL NO. 2

2.2 VISHAKTA AHARA PARIKSHA

Experiment

7. Detection of Adulteration in PANEER

Aim:

Principle:

Materials:

Procedure:

Observation:

Result:

Teacher Signature

DETECTION OF ADULTERATION IN PANEER AS PER FSSAI GUIDELINES

fssai
FOOD SAFETY AND STANDARDS AUTHORITY OF INDIA

Paneer is a milk product. It may be adulterated with starch, vegetable fat, neutralizers, detergents, urea or synthetic milk. The following tests are prescribed as per FSSAI guidelines to detect common adulterants in paneer.

Principle:
Adulterants give specific chemical reactions with reagents which produce characteristic colour change or precipitate.

REQUIREMENTS

- Fresh paneer sample
- Distilled water
- Iodine solution (0.1 N)
- Concentrated HCl
- Fehling's Solution A & B
- Sodium hydroxide (NaOH)
- Copper sulphate solution (1%)
- Chloroform
- Filter paper, Test tubes, Glass rod, Droppers

SAMPLE PREPARATION

Grind 10 g of paneer and add 20 ml of distilled water.
Shake well and filter.
Use the filtrate for different tests.

PROCEDURE

1 TEST FOR STARCH

Take 2 ml of sample filtrate in a test tube.
Add 2–3 drops of iodine solution.

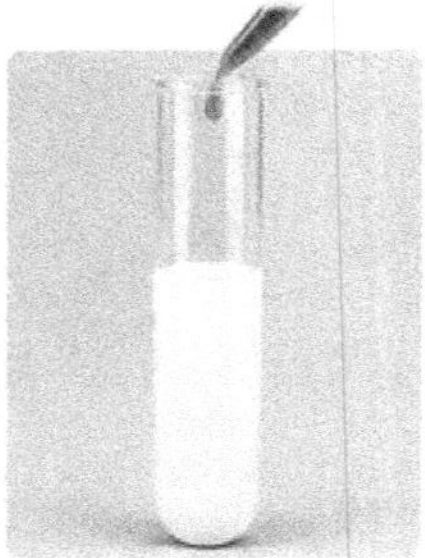

Blue colour indicates starch

2 TEST FOR NEUTRALIZERS
(Added to correct excess acidity)

Take 2 ml of sample filtrate. Add 2–3 drops of phenolphthalein solution and then add NaOH dropwise.

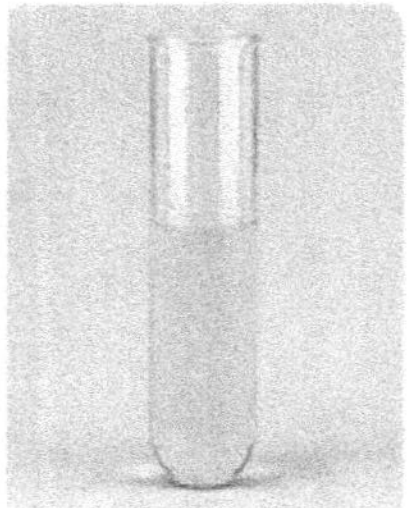

Pink colour indicates presence of neutralizers

3 TEST FOR SUGAR
(Added for sweetness)

Take 2 ml of sample filtrate. Add equal amount of Fehling's Solution A & B.
Boil for 2 minutes.

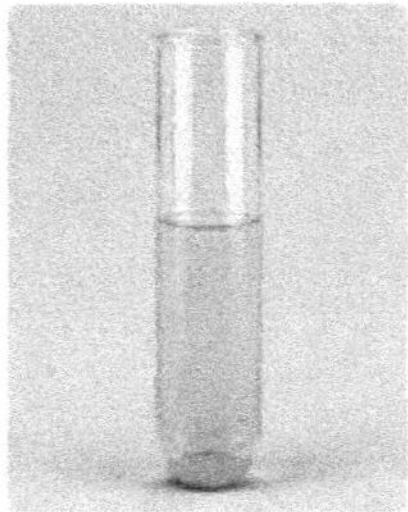

Brick red precipitate indicates presence of sugar

4 TEST FOR UREA

Take 2 ml of sample filtrate. Add 1 ml of Coper sulphate solution and then 1 ml of NaOH solution.

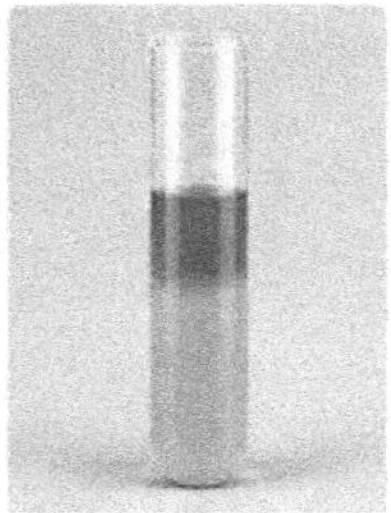

Pink / violet colour indicates presence of urea

5 TEST FOR DETERGENTS

Take 5 ml of sample filtrate in a test tube.
Shake well after adding a few drops of chloroform.

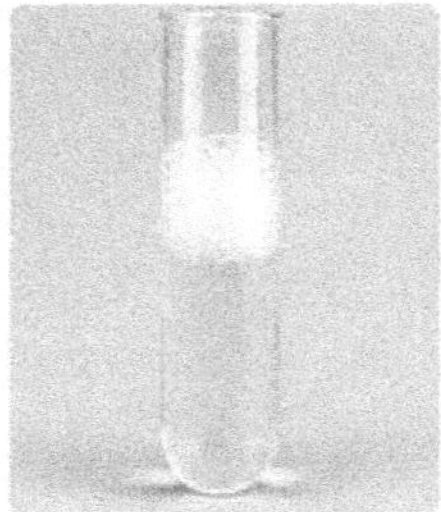

Persistent froth indicates presence of detergents

6 TEST FOR FOREIGN FAT / VEGETABLE FAT

Boil a small piece of paneer with few ml of water. Filter and add few drops of HCl.

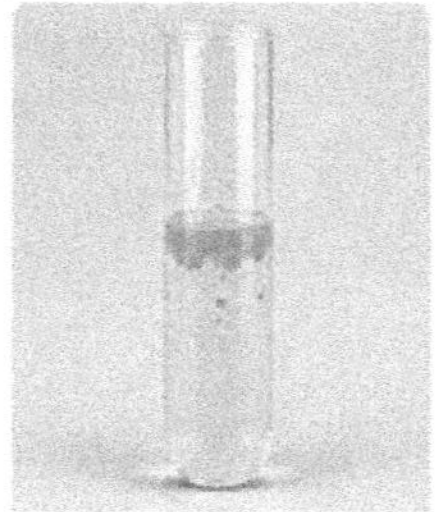

Red / orange colour floating layer indicates foreign fat / vegetable fat

OBSERVATION AND INFERENCE

Test	Observation	Inference (Adulteration)
Starch Test	Blue or blue-black colour	Presence of starch
Neutralizer Test	Pink colour	Presence of neutralizers (e.g., Na_2CO_3, $NaHCO_3$)
Sugar Test	Brick red precipitate	Presence of added sugar
Urea Test	Pink / violet colour	Presence of urea
Detergent Test	Persistent froth	Presence of detergents
Foreign Fat Test	Red / orange coloured layer	Presence of foreign fat / vegetable fat

NOTES

- Adulteration is not permitted as per FSSAI standards.
- Presence of adulterants affects quality and is hazardous to health.
- These are qualitative tests. For confirmation and quantification, instrumental methods like HPLC, GC-MS, FTIR may be used.
- Always use fresh reagents and clean glassware.

FSSAI LIMIT (General)

Parameter	Permitted Level
Starch	Not Permitted
Urea	Not Permitted
Detergents	Not Permitted
Neutralizers	Not Permitted
Foreign Fat	Not Permitted
Added Sugar	Not Permitted

PRECAUTIONS

- Use fresh paneer sample.
- Use clean and dry test tubes.
- Do not mix reagents with mouth.
- Perform tests in a clean environment.

CONCLUSION

The above tests help in the detection of common adulterants in paneer as per FSSAI guidelines and ensure safety, quality and purity of the food for consumers.

REFERENCE

FSSAI Manual of Methods of Analysis of Foods, 1st Edition, 2015, Methods: 1.7.2, 1.7.4, 1.7.6, 1.7.7, 1.7.8, 1.7.10

DIAGNOSIS AND MANAGEMENT OF DISEASES DUE TO GARAVISHA, DOOSHIVISHA AND VISHA UPADRAVA

Visha Chikitsa OPD

DRUG INDUCED TOXICITIES

Forensic Science For Justice

1. GARAVISHA

Poison formed by improper processing, preparation or storage of drugs or food. It acts slowly and produces chronic diseases.

CAUSES

- Improper harvesting, processing or storage of drugs/food
- Use of unclean vessels, contaminated water
- Adulteration and wrong combination
- Violation of pharmaceutical procedures

FEATURES

- Long latent period
- Insidious onset
- Chronic disease picture
- Mild but persistent symptoms

DIAGNOSIS

- Detailed history of diet, drugs and habits
- Clinical examination
- Examination of tongue, stool, urine
- Laboratory investigations (Hb%, LFT, RFT etc.)

MANAGEMENT

General Principles

- ✓ Nidana Parivarjana (avoid causative factors)
- ✓ Shodhana (Vamana, Virechana as indicated)
- ✓ Shamana (Medhya, Rasayana, Deepana, Pachana)
- ✓ Pathyapathya (appropriate diet and regimen)

USEFUL YOGAS

- Panchakola Churna
- Chitrakadi Vati
- Arogya Vardhini Vati
- Guduchi, Haridra, Amalaki

2. DOOSHIVISHA

Poison produced in the body due to vitiation of Doshas by improper diet, lifestyle, environment and mental factors.

Vata
Pitta
Kapha

CAUSES

- Viruddha Ahara (incompatible diet)
- Atyashana (overeating) or Alpa Ahara (undereating)
- Adhyashana (eating before digestion of previous food)
- Mithya Ahara Vihara (improper regimen)
- Suppression of natural urges
- Mental factors – stress, anger, grief etc.

FEATURES

- Symptoms due to vitiation of Doshas
- Affects Srotas and Dhatus
- Manifest as various systemic disorders

DIAGNOSIS

- History of diet, regimen and mental factors
- Clinical features according to dosha predominance
- Dashavidha Pariksha (10 fold examination)
- Lab investigations as per need

MANAGEMENT

General Principles

- ✓ Nidana Parivarjana
- ✓ Shodhana (Panchakarma as indicated)
- ✓ Shamana (Deepana, Pachana, Srotoshodhana)
- ✓ Pathya Ahara Vihara
- ✓ Rasayana (to restore balance)

USEFUL YOGAS

- Triphala Churna
- Avipattikara Churna
- Guduchi Satva
- Panchatikta Ghrita Guggulu

3. VISHA UPADRAVA

Complications arising due to spread of poison in the body or due to improper management of poisoning. It may be early or late.

TYPES

- Early Upadrava – during the course of poisoning
- Late Upadrava – after some time
- Site-specific complications – organ or system involvement

CLINICAL FEATURES (Examples)

- Jwara, Atisara, Chardi
- Daha, Daha Praseka
- Murchha, Bhrama
- Kushta, Kamala
- Shotha, Hrillasa
- Organ dysfunction, failure

DIAGNOSIS

- Detailed history of poisoning
- Clinical examination
- Investigations (CBC, RFT, LFT, ECG, X-ray etc.)
- Rule out complications

MANAGEMENT

- ✓ Treat the primary poisoning
- ✓ Supportive therapy
- ✓ Specific management of complications
- ✓ Rasayana and Basti in chronic cases
- ✓ Diet and lifestyle correction

USEFUL YOGAS

- Mrityunjaya Rasa
- Sanjeevani Vati
- Punarnavadi Kwatha
- Yashtimadhu, Guduchi

DRUG INDUCED TOXICITIES – OVERVIEW

GENERAL POINTS

- Drug induced toxicity is a type of Dooshivisha.
- Can occur due to overdose, prolonged use, drug interactions or hypersensitivity.
- Affects any organ or system.
- Early recognition and proper management prevents complications.

COMMON ORGANS AFFECTED

- Liver (Hepatotoxicity)
- Kidney (Nephrotoxicity)
- Heart (Cardiotoxicity)
- Nervous System (Neurotoxicity)
- Skin (Dermatotoxicity)
- Blood (Hematotoxicity)
- Gastrointestinal Tract (GI Toxicity)

CAUSES

- Overdose
- Prolonged use
- Drug interactions
- Allergic / Hypersensitivity reactions
- Wrong route / Wrong dose / Wrong patient

CLINICAL FEATURES (General)

- Nausea, vomiting
- Loss of appetite
- Weakness, fatigue
- Headache, dizziness
- Skin rashes, itching
- Abdominal pain
- Jaundice
- Breathlessness, palpitations
- Altered sensorium / Convulsions
- Organ dysfunction / failure

MANAGEMENT PRINCIPLES

STEP	MANAGEMENT	EXAMPLES / NOTES
1.Stop the offending drug	Immediate withdrawal of the causative drug.	Most important first step.
2.Assessment	History, clinical examination, vital signs and investigations.	CBC, LFT, RFT, ECG, etc.
3.Decontamination (if early)	Vamana, Virechana, Activated charcoal (as applicable).	As per time and type of toxicity.
4.Supportive care	IV fluids, O_2 support, correction of electrolytes.	Maintain vitals and organ function.
5.Specific management	Treat based on organ/system affected.	Hepatoprotectives, nephroprotectives, etc.
6.Shamana therapy	Deepana, Pachana, Srotoshodhana, Rasayana.	Herbal formulations as per condition.
7.Pathya & Vihara	Appropriate diet, rest, and avoidance of causative factors.	Essential for complete recovery.
8.Follow up	Regular monitoring and review of investigations.	Prevent recurrence and complications.

AYURVEDIC SUPPORTIVE DRUGS

- Guduchi - Immunomodulator, hepatoprotective
- Haridra - Anti-inflammatory, antioxidant
- Yashtimadhu - Soothing, antiulcer
- Bhringaraja - Hepatoprotective
- Punarnava - Diuretic, nephroprotective
- Amalaki - Rasayana, antioxidant
- Triphala - Detoxifying, antioxidant

DO'S

- Use drugs in proper dose and duration.
- Check drug interactions.
- Monitor patients on long term drugs.
- Report adverse drug reactions.
- Maintain good documentation.

DON'TS

- Do not self-medicate.
- Do not exceed prescribed dose.
- Do not ignore early symptoms.
- Do not use expired / adulterated drugs.
- Do not mix incompatible drugs.

"Right drug, right dose, right patient, right time – the essence of safe therapy."

Dr Anil Kumar Y
Assistant Professor
Department of Agada Tantra (Visha Chikitsa OPD)
TMAE's Ayurveda Medical College & Hospital, Hospete

Visha Vaidya

"Ayurveda teaches us to treat the cause, protect the body, and promote holistic healing."

PRACTICAL NO. 3

DOOSHIVISHA / GARAVISHA CASE RECORD

Drug Induced toxicity

Case No:01

Date:

Patient Details

Name::

Age::

Sex:

Address:

Occupation:

Chief Complaints:

History of Present Illness:

Exposure History:

Nidana:

Examination:

Samprapti:

Differential Diagnosis:

Diagnosis:

Treatment Given

Outcome

Discussion

Faculty Signature

DIAGNOSIS AND MANAGEMENT OF DISEASES DUE TO GARAVISHA, DOOSHIVISHA AND VISHA UPADRAVA

Visha Chikitsa OPD

OCCUPATIONAL HAZARDS

Forensic Science For Justice

- **Garavisha** – Poison formed due to improper processing, storage or combination of drugs/chemicals.
- **Dooshivisha** – Poison accumulated in the body due to long term exposure to low dose toxins in occupation.
- **Visha Upadrava** – Complications arising from acute or chronic exposure to occupational toxins.

OCCUPATIONAL HAZARDS – COMMON SOURCES

Industrial Chemicals | Heavy Metals | Pesticides & Herbicides | Solvents & Fumes | Dusts & Fibers | Biomedical Waste | Radiation

1. GARAVISHA – OCCUPATIONAL EXPOSURE

COMMON OCCUPATIONS

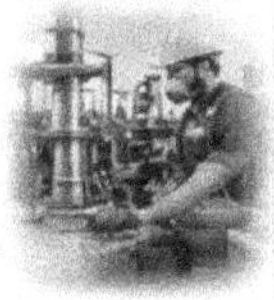

- Workers in chemical industries, refineries
- Paint and varnish manufacturers
- Battery, plastic and rubber industries
- Cleaning staff (exposure to disinfectants)
- Laboratory technicians handling reagents

CAUSES

- Exposure to processed or concentrated chemicals
- Improper handling of toxic substances
- Inhalation, ingestion or skin contact

CLINICAL FEATURES

- Headache
- Nausea, vomiting
- Giddiness
- Skin irritation, rashes
- Breathlessness
- Weakness, fatigue

DIAGNOSIS

- Detailed occupational history
- Clinical examination
- Lab investigations (CBC, LFT, RFT, Urine routine, Toxicology)
- Specific tests (Blood/urine heavy metals, Pesticide levels)

MANAGEMENT

- ✓ Immediate removal from exposure
- ✓ Nidana Parivarjana
- ✓ Shodhana (Vamana/Virechana as indicated)
- ✓ Shamana with appropriate formulations
- ✓ Supportive care, hydration and nutrition

USEFUL YOGAS

- Guduchi, Haridra, Amalaki
- Pancha Tikta Ghrita Guggulu
- Nimba, Manjishta, Triphala

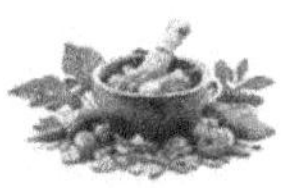

2. DOOSHIVISHA – OCCUPATIONAL EXPOSURE

COMMON OCCUPATIONS

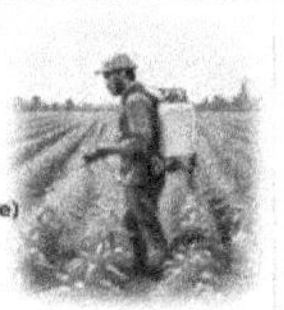

- Pesticide applicators and farmers
- Miners and smelter workers
- Workers in dye, textile, tannery
- Health care workers (long term exposure)
- E-waste handlers

CAUSES

- Chronic low dose exposure to toxins
- Accumulation of toxins in body (Dosha Dushti)
- Improper diet, lifestyle and inadequate detox

CLINICAL FEATURES

- Loss of appetite
- Indigestion
- Skin diders
- Joint pain
- Generalized weakness
- Mental irritability

DIAGNOSIS

- Detailed occupational and dietary history
- Clinical examination
- Lab investigations (LFT, RFT, CBC, Urine routine)
- Specific tests (Heavy metals, Pesticide residue etc.)

MANAGEMENT

- ✓ Nidana Parivarjana (avoid further exposure)
- ✓ Shodhana (Virechana, Basti, Raktamokshana if needed)
- ✓ Rasayana (Amalaki, Guduchi, Haritaki)
- ✓ Pathya-Apathya and lifestyle correction

USEFUL YOGAS

- Guduchi Satva
- Triphala Churna
- Panchakarma (as per need)
- Rasayana Churna

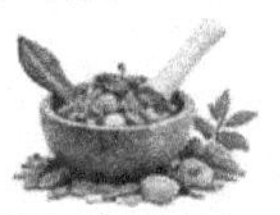

3. VISHA UPADRAVA – OCCUPATIONAL COMPLICATIONS

COMMON OCCUPATIONS

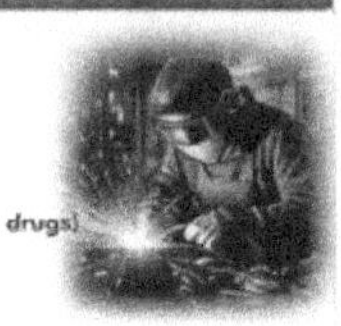

- Welders (fume exposure)
- Construction workers (silica dust)
- Radiology staff (radiation exposure)
- Health care workers (needle stick, cytotoxic drugs)
- Workers in foundries and glass industries

TYPES OF UPADRAVA

- Early Upadrava – headache, irritation, mild symptoms
- Late Upadrava – organ/system involvement
- Site specific – respiratory, skin, neurological, renal etc.

CLINICAL FEATURES (Examples)

- Respiratory complaints
- Dermatitis, ulcers
- Neurological symptoms
- Hepatic / Renal dysfunction
- Anemia
- Reproductive problems

DIAGNOSIS

- Detailed history and clinical examination
- Organ specific investigations (PFT, X-ray, USG, ECG etc.)
- Toxicology tests, Biopsy (if indicated)
- Assessment of severity and complications

MANAGEMENT

- ✓ Remove from exposure and stabilize
- ✓ Treat according to organ/system involved
- ✓ Specific antidotes if available
- ✓ Rasayana and restorative therapy
- ✓ Rehabilitation and follow up

USEFUL YOGAS

- Punarnava Mandura
- Bhringaraja, Kalmegha
- Yashtimadhu, Guduchi
- Chyavanaprasha, Brahmi

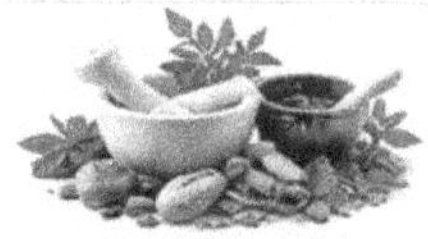

COMMON OCCUPATIONAL TOXICITIES – EXAMPLES

TOXIN / AGENT	SOURCES / OCCUPATION	EFFECTS	INVESTIGATIONS
Lead	Battery, paint, plumbing	Anemia, abdominal colic, neurotoxicity	Blood lead level, CBC
Mercury	Thermometer, electrical, mining	Tremors, gingivitis, renal damage	Blood/urine mercury
Cadmium	Batteries, pigments, welding	Kidney damage, bone demineralization	Urine cadmium
Pesticides (OP)	Agriculture, pest control	Nausea, salivation, muscle weakness	Cholinesterase level
Solvents (Benzene, Toluene)	Paint, adhesive, printing	Headache, dizziness, leukemia (chronic)	CBC, LFT
Silica Dust	Construction, mining	Silicosis, TB, lung fibrosis	X-ray chest, PFT
Radiation	Radiology, nuclear industry	Burns, cancer, infertility	Dose assessment, CBC

GENERAL MANAGEMENT PRINCIPLES

1. Early recognition and removal from exposure
2. Supportive and symptomatic treatment
3. Detoxification (Shodhana) based on condition
4. Use of appropriate Ayurvedic formulations
5. Diet, lifestyle modification and Rasayana
6. Regular monitoring and follow up

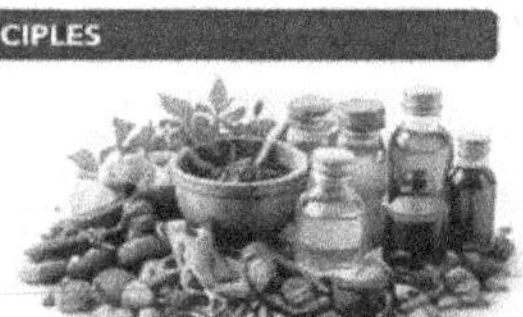

PREVENTIVE MEASURES

- Use of Personal Protective Equipment (PPE)
- Proper ventilation and safety measures
- Safe storage and handling of chemicals
- Regular health check-up of workers
- Awareness and training programs
- Immediate reporting of exposure incidents

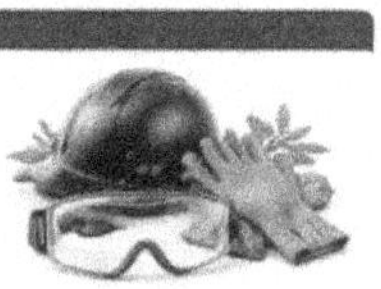

DO's AND DON'Ts

DO's

- Follow safety protocols strictly.
- Use PPEs at workplace.
- Maintain personal and workplace hygiene.
- Drink plenty of water and eat balanced diet.
- Report early symptoms to medical officer.

DON'Ts

- Do not ignore safety instructions.
- Do not mix chemicals or use expired substances.
- Do not eat or smoke in hazardous areas.
- Do not delay treatment.

PATHYA – APATHYA (GENERAL)

PATHYA	APATHYA
Light, easily digestible food	Junk food, heavy meals
Fresh fruits, green vegetables	Alcohol, smoking
Amalaki, Guduchi, Nimba	Excessive spicy, oily food
Adequate sleep and rest	Irregular sleep and routines
Stress management	Re-exposure to toxins

REMEMBER

"Protection at work today ensures a healthy life tomorrow."

Scan for Learning Videos and Resources

Visha Vaidya

Dr Anil Kumar Y
Assistant Professor
Department of Agada Tantra (Visha Chikitsa OPD)
TMAE's Ayurveda Medical College & Hospital, Hospete

"Ayurveda protects the body from poison, preserves health and promotes longevity."

PRACTICAL NO. 3

DOOSHIVISHA / GARAVISHA CASE RECORD

Occupational Hazards

Case No:02

Date:

Patient Details

Name::

Age::

Sex:

Address:

Occupation:

Chief Complaints:

History of Present Illness:

Exposure History:

Nidana:

Examination:

Samprapti:

Differential Diagnosis:

Diagnosis:

Treatment Given

Outcome

Discussion

Faculty Signature

Visha Chikitsa OPD

DIAGNOSIS AND MANAGEMENT OF DISEASES DUE TO GARAVISHA, DOOSHIVISHA AND VISHA UPADRAVA

ALLERGIC MANIFESTATIONS

Forensic Science For Justice

Allergic manifestations can occur due to intake, contact, inhalation or parenteral exposure to allergens or toxins. Ayurveda explains these conditions under the spectrum of Dooshivisha and Visha Upadrava.

1. GARAVISHA – ALLERGIC MANIFESTATIONS

Allergic reactions caused by incompatibility of food, drugs or medicinal preparations with the body (Garavisha).

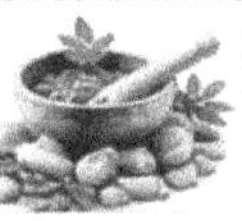

CAUSES

- Viruddha Ahara (incompatible food combinations)
- Adhyashana (overeating)
- Improper digestion of previous food
- Chemical additives, preservatives in food
- Self medication and overuse of drugs

CLINICAL FEATURES

- Urticaria (Shitapitta)
- Nausea, vomiting
- Itching (Kandu)
- Loose stools
- Skin rashes, redness
- Breathlessness (in severe cases)

DIAGNOSIS

- Detailed history of diet and drug intake
- Clinical examination of skin and systemic involvement
- Investigations: CBC (eosinophilia), LFT, RFT, Serum IgE (if needed)
- Allergy testing (Skin prick test / Specific IgE)

MANAGEMENT

- ✓ Nidana Parivarjana (avoid causative factors)
- ✓ Shodhana (Vamana / Virechana as indicated)
- ✓ Shamana (Antihistaminic, Tikta, Kashaya drugs)
- ✓ Pathya-Apathya and lifestyle correction

USEFUL YOGAS

- Panchatikta Ghrita Guggulu
- Gandhaka Rasayana
- Avipattikara Churna
- Sutashekhara Rasa (as indicated)

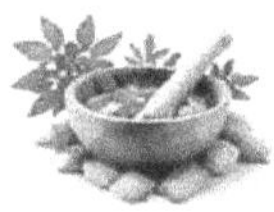

2. DOOSHIVISHA – ALLERGIC MANIFESTATIONS

Allergic manifestations due to long term exposure to low dose toxins, drugs, chemicals or environmental pollutants.

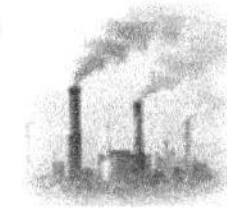

CAUSES

- Chronic exposure to pesticides, heavy metals, chemicals
- Occupational exposure (industrial, agricultural)
- Continued intake of low quality food and additives
- Environmental pollution (air, water, soil)

CLINICAL FEATURES

- Chronic urticaria
- Watery eyes, sneezing
- Eczema / Dermatitis
- Headache, fatigue
- Recurrent respiratory allergies (Rhinitis, Asthma)
- Gastrointestinal complaints

DIAGNOSIS

- Detailed exposure history (occupation, environment)
- Clinical examination
- Investigations: CBC (eosinophilia), IgE, PFT (in respiratory allergy), LFT, RFT
- Allergy testing, Patch test (if indicated)

MANAGEMENT

- ✓ Nidana Parivarjana (avoid exposure)
- ✓ Rasayana and immunity enhancers
- ✓ Shodhana (Virechana / Basti as per condition)
- ✓ Shamana (Tikta, Raktashodhaka, Deepana drugs)

USEFUL YOGAS

- Khadirarishta
- Mahamanjishtadi Kashaya
- Guduchi Satva
- Panchatikta Ghrita

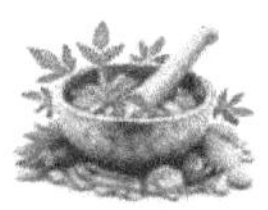

3. VISHA UPADRAVA – ALLERGIC MANIFESTATIONS

Complications arising due to acute or chronic poisoning leading to allergic or hypersensitivity reactions.

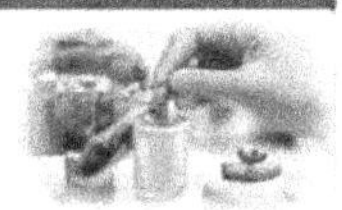

TYPES

- Early Upadrava – appear soon after exposure (minutes to hours)
- Late Upadrava – appear after some time (days to weeks)
- Severe systemic reactions – Anaphylaxis

CLINICAL FEATURES (Examples)

- Anaphylaxis (Severe itching, hives, swelling, hypotension)
- Stevens-Johnson syndrome
- Angioedema (swelling of face, lips, eyelids)
- Drug eruptions (Maculopapular, Erythema, Blistering)
- Bronchospasm (wheezing, dyspnea)
- Systemic involvement (Fever, weakness)

DIAGNOSIS

- Detailed history of exposure and onset
- Clinical examination for severity and system involvement
- Investigations: CBC, LFT, RFT, Serum tryptase (if anaphylaxis suspected), ABG, ECG
- Skin / Patch / Provocation test (if required)

MANAGEMENT

- ✓ Immediate management of acute poisoning
- ✓ Emergency care (Airway, Breathing, Circulation)
- ✓ Antihistaminics, Corticosteroids, Adrenaline (in anaphylaxis)
- ✓ Rasayana and supportive therapy for recovery

USEFUL YOGAS

- Mrityunjaya Rasa
- Sanjeevani Vati
- Yashtimadhu Ghrita
- Pushkarmoola Asava

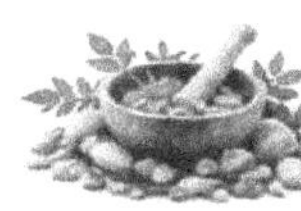

COMPARISON OF ALLERGIC MANIFESTATIONS

FEATURES	GARAVISHA	DOOSHIVISHA	VISHA UPADRAVA
Nature	Due to incompatible food/drug combinations	Due to long term low dose exposure	Due to acute/chronic poisoning
Onset	Early (hours to a few days)	Insidious (weeks to months)	Early or late (based on poison and dose)
Duration	Usually acute and self-limiting	Chronic, recurrent	Varies – acute/severe or chronic
Clinical Features	Itching, rashes, urticaria, GI upset	Chronic skin, respiratory & systemic symptoms	Severe allergic reactions, systemic involvement
Diagnosis	Diet/drug history, clinical, basic labs	Exposure history, labs, allergy tests	History of poisoning, severity assessment, labs
Management	Avoid cause, shodhana, shamana	Avoid exposure, rasayana, shodhana, shamana	Emergency care, specific treatment, support

MANAGEMENT

- **NIDANA PARIVARJANA** – Avoid causative food, drugs, chemicals, occupational and environmental exposures.
- **SHODHANA CHIKITSA** – Vamana (emesis), Virechana (purgation), Basti (medicated enema) as per indication.
- **SHAMANA CHIKITSA** – Use of Tikta (bitter), Kashaya (astringent), Raktashodhaka (blood purifiers), Deepana-Pachana drugs.
- **RASAYANA CHIKITSA** – Strengthen immunity and promote tissue healing (Guduchi, Amalaki, Haridra etc.).
- **PATHYA – APATHYA** – Light, easily digestible diet, proper sleep, stress management, clean environment.

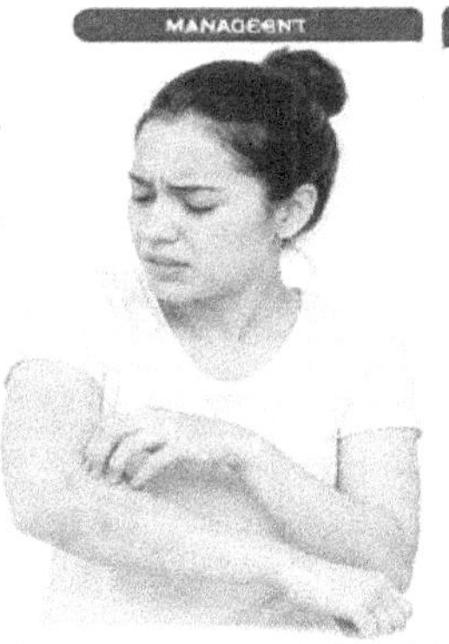

IMPORTANT AYURVEDIC DRUGS

Raktashodhaka & Allergy Pacifiers: Guduchi, Nimba, Manjishta, Haridra, Khadira, Guggulu

Immunomodulators & Rasayana: Amalaki, Ashwagandha, Shatavari, Yashtimadhu, Guduchi Satva, Chyavanprasha

Other Useful Drugs (As per Indication): Avipattikara Churna, Panchatikta Ghrita, Sutashekhara Rasa, Mrityunjaya Rasa, Sanjeevani Vati, Mahamanjishtadi Kashaya

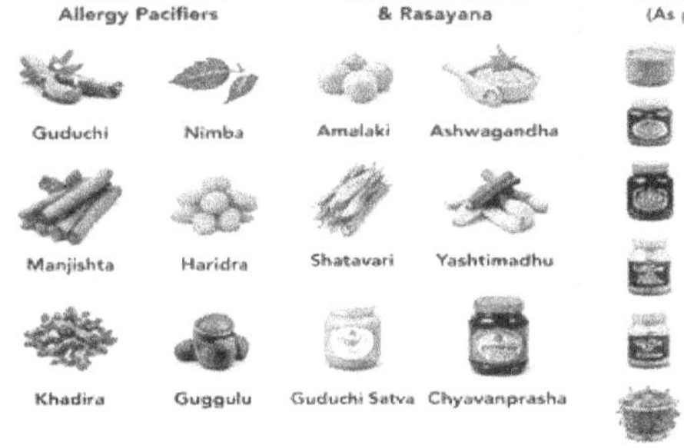

DO'S

- Take medicines as prescribed
- Avoid self medication
- Follow a light, wholesome diet
- Maintain personal and occupational hygiene
- Report early symptoms to doctor

DON'TS

- Do not ignore early symptoms
- Do not re-expose to the allergen/toxin
- Do not take incompatible food/drugs
- Do not overuse or misuse medicines
- Do not consume junk and processed food

ALLERGIC EMERGENCY – DO THIS

- Stop exposure immediately
- Give first aid and supportive care
- Administer emergency drugs (Adrenaline, Antihistamines, Steroids) as needed
- Shift to hospital without delay

REMEMBER

"Identify early, avoid the cause, treat wisely and restore balance – that is the key to recovery from allergic manifestations."

Scan for Learning Videos & Resources

Visha Vaidya

Dr Anil Kumar Y
Assistant Professor
Department of Agada Tantra (Visha Chikitsa OPD)
TMAE's Ayurveda Medical College & Hospital, Hospete

"Ayurveda heals not just the disease, but the root cause and restores harmony."

PRACTICAL NO. 3

DOOSHIVISHA / GARAVISHA CASE RECORD

Allergic Manifestations

Case No:03

Date:

Patient Details

Name::

Age::

Sex:

Address:

Occupation:

Chief Complaints:

History of Present Illness:

Exposure History:

Nidana:

Examination:

Samprapti:

Differential Diagnosis:

Diagnosis:

Treatment Given

Outcome

Discussion

Faculty Signature

DIAGNOSIS AND MANAGEMENT OF DISEASES DUE TO
GARAVISHA, DOOSHIVISHA AND VISHA UPADRAVA

Visha Chikitsa OPD

Forensic Science For Justice

AUTOIMMUNE DISEASES – AN AYURVEDIC PERSPECTIVE

Autoimmune diseases arise when the body's immune system mistakenly attacks its own tissues. In Ayurveda, they can be understood as a result of vitiation of Doshas, especially Vata and Pitta, vitiated Rakta (blood), Dhatus and Agni, due to the action of Garavisha (accumulated toxic load), Dooshivisha (low grade toxins) and Visha Upadrava (complications of toxins).

1. GARAVISHA – AUTOIMMUNE DISEASES

Accumulation of heavy, potent toxins (Garavisha) in the body over a long period due to improper diet, drugs, chemicals, heavy metals, pollutants etc. These toxins lodge in Dhatus and cause deep seated immune dysregulation.

CAUSES

- Long term intake of incompatible food
- Excessive use of allopathic drugs (steroids, immunosuppressants)
- Exposure to heavy metals, pesticides, industrial chemicals
- Adverse environmental conditions

CLINICAL FEATURES

- Chronic fatigue
- Organ specific inflammation
- Joint pain & stiffness
- Low grade fever
- Rashes / Urticaria
- Dhatu kshaya (tissue wasting)

EXAMPLES OF DISEASES

- Rheumatoid arthritis, Systemic lupus erythematosus (SLE), Psoriasis, Multiple sclerosis, Type 1 diabetes mellitus, Autoimmune thyroiditis etc.

DIAGNOSIS

- Detailed history of diet, drug & toxin exposure
- Clinical features & autoimmune markers (ANA, RF, Anti-dsDNA etc.)
- Investigations: CBC, ESR, CRP, Autoantibodies, Organ function tests

MANAGEMENT

- ✓ Nidana Parivarjana – avoid causative factors
- ✓ Shodhana (Virechana, Basti) to expel toxins
- ✓ Shamana with Rasayana & Deepana-Pachana
- ✓ Immunomodulation & Dhatu poshana

USEFUL YOGAS

- Panchatikta Ghrita Guggulu
- Maharasnadi Kashaya
- Guduchi Satva

2. DOOSHIVISHA – AUTOIMMUNE DISEASES

Low grade toxins produced within the body or introduced through diet, lifestyle, infections, emotional stress etc. These toxins gradually accumulate and disturb immune tolerance.

CAUSES

- Improper diet & eating habits
- Ama formation due to Mandagni
- Chronic infections & poor gut health
- Stress, lack of sleep, sedentary lifestyle

CLINICAL FEATURES

- Bloating, heaviness
- Mild pain in joints
- Irregular bowel habits
- Food senstivities
- Skin disorders
- Recurrent infections

EXAMPLES OF DISEASES

- Hashimoto's thyroiditis, Ulcerative colitis, Vitiligo, Alopecia areata, Psoriasis, Irritable bowel syndrome with autoimmunity.

DIAGNOSIS

- Detailed diet & lifestyle history
- Clinical examination & autoimmune markers
- Investigations: CBC, ESR, CRP, ANA, TSH, etc.

MANAGEMENT

- ✓ Deepana-Pachana to correct Agni & Ama
- ✓ Shodhana (Vamana, Virechana, Basti as indicated)
- ✓ Shamana with Tikta, Katu, Kashaya dravyas
- ✓ Diet & lifestyle correction, stress management

USEFUL YOGAS

- Triphala Guggulu
- Kanchanara Guggulu
- Avipattikara Churna

3. VISHA UPADRAVA – AUTOIMMUNE DISEASES

Complications arising from spread of toxins (Visha) in the body or due to improper management of poisoning. It causes immune imbalance and tissue damage.

TYPES

- Early Upadrava – mild immune dysregulation
- Late Upadrava – chronic autoimmune disorders
- Site specific – organ or system involvement

CLINICAL FEATURES (Examples)

- Severe inflammation
- Vasculitis
- Organ dysfunction
- Renal involvement
- Neurological symptoms
- Hematological disorders

EXAMPLES OF DISEASES

- Vasculitis, Autoimmune hepatitis, Autoimmune encephalitis, Myasthenia gravis, Goodpasture syndrome, Dermatomyositis.

DIAGNOSIS

- History of poisoning / toxin exposure
- Systemic examination & autoimmune profile
- Investigations: ANA, ANCA, LFT, KFT, MRI, Biopsy

MANAGEMENT

- ✓ Treat the underlying toxin exposure
- ✓ Shodhana to eliminate toxins
- ✓ Rasayana & Balya for tissue repair
- ✓ Supportive & organ specific management

USEFUL YOGAS

- Maharasnadi Kashaya
- Punarnavadi Kwatha
- Punarnavadi Kwatha

COMPARISON OF GARAVISHA, DOOSHIVISHA & VISHA UPADRAVA IN AUTOIMMUNE DISEASES

FEATURES	GARAVISHA	DOOSHIVISHA	VISHA UPADRAVA
Nature	Accumulated potent toxins (heavy, stable)	Low grade toxins (viral, metabolic, environmental)	Complications of toxins or poisoning
Origin	External (drugs, chemicals, heavy metals, environment)	Internal & external (diet, ama, infections, stress)	Spread of toxins within body
Duration	Long standing (years)	Insidious (months to years)	Acute to chronic (varies)
Onset	Slow and progressive	Gradual and recurrent	May be sudden or gradual
Dosha Involvement	Vata-Pitta pradhana with Rakta dushti	Kapha-Pitta with Ama	Tridosha with Rakta, Srotodushti
Dhatu Involvement	Deep dhatu involvement (Mamsa, Asthi, Majja)	Rasa, Rakta, Mamsa	Specific organ/system involvement
Example Diseases	RA, SLE, MS, Psoriasis, Type 1 DM	Hashimoto's, UC, Vitiligo, Alopecia	Vasculitis, Autoimmune hepatitis, MG
Management Focus	Toxin elimination + Rasayana + Immunomodulation	Ama pachana + Agni deepana + Lifestyle correction	Treat complication + Organ support

PATHOGENESIS (SAMPRAPTI) IN AUTOIMMUNE DISEASES

Nidana Sevana (toxic exposure, improper diet, stress)
↓
Dosha Prakopa (Vata, Pitta, Kapha)
↓
Ama & Dooshivisha / Garavisha formation
↓
Srotorodha & Dhatu Dushti
↓
Rakta Dushti & Immune Dysregulation
↓
Autoimmune Response
↓
Tissue Damage & Clinical Disease

IMPORTANT AYURVEDIC PRINCIPLES

1. Nidana Parivarjana – Avoid toxins, incompatible food & stress
2. Agni Deepana & Ama Pachana – Correct metabolic fire
3. Shodhana – Eliminate accumulated toxins
4. Shamana – Pacify Doshas & modulate immunity
5. Rasayana – Rejuvenate & repair tissues
6. Pathya - Apatya – Follow suitable diet & lifestyle
7. Manasika Chikitsa – Stress management, meditation, yoga

AYURVEDIC SUPPORTIVE DRUGS

Guduchi, Nimba, Haridra, Ashwagandha, Amalaki, Shallaki, Manjistha, Yashtimadhu, Brahmi, Guggulu, Punarnava, Triphala

DO'S

- Follow Pathya Ahara & Vihara
- Take medicines on time
- Practice Yoga, Pranayama & Meditation
- Maintain gut health & regular bowel habits
- Avoid self medication & suppressive therapy

DON'TS

- Do not consume incompatible food
- Do not overuse steroids & immunosuppressants
- Do not ignore early symptoms
- Do not expose to chemicals/pollutants
- Do not neglect sleep & stress

YOGA & LIFESTYLE

Nadi Shodhana, Bhramari, Setu Bandhasana, Shavasana

- Regular exercise, adequate sleep
- Avoid excessive work & mental stress
- Practice mindfulness & positive thinking

REMEMBER

"Balance of Agni, purity of Dhatus and a calm mind restore immune harmony."

Scan for Learning Videos & Resources

Visha Vaidya

Dr Anil Kumar Y
Assistant Professor
Department of Agada Tantra (Visha Chikitsa OPD)
TMAE's Ayurveda Medical College & Hospital, Hospete

"Ayurveda does not suppress the immunity; it corrects the cause and restores balance."

"Ayurveda teaches us to eliminate the toxin, balance the immunity and promote holistic healing."

PRACTICAL NO. 3

DOOSHIVISHA / GARAVISHA CASE RECORD

Autoimmune Diseases

Case No:04

Date:

Patient Details

Name::

Age::

Sex:

Address:

Occupation:

Chief Complaints:

History of Present Illness:

Exposure History:

Nidana:

Examination:

Samprapti:

Differential Diagnosis:

Diagnosis:

Treatment Given

Outcome

Discussion

Faculty Signature

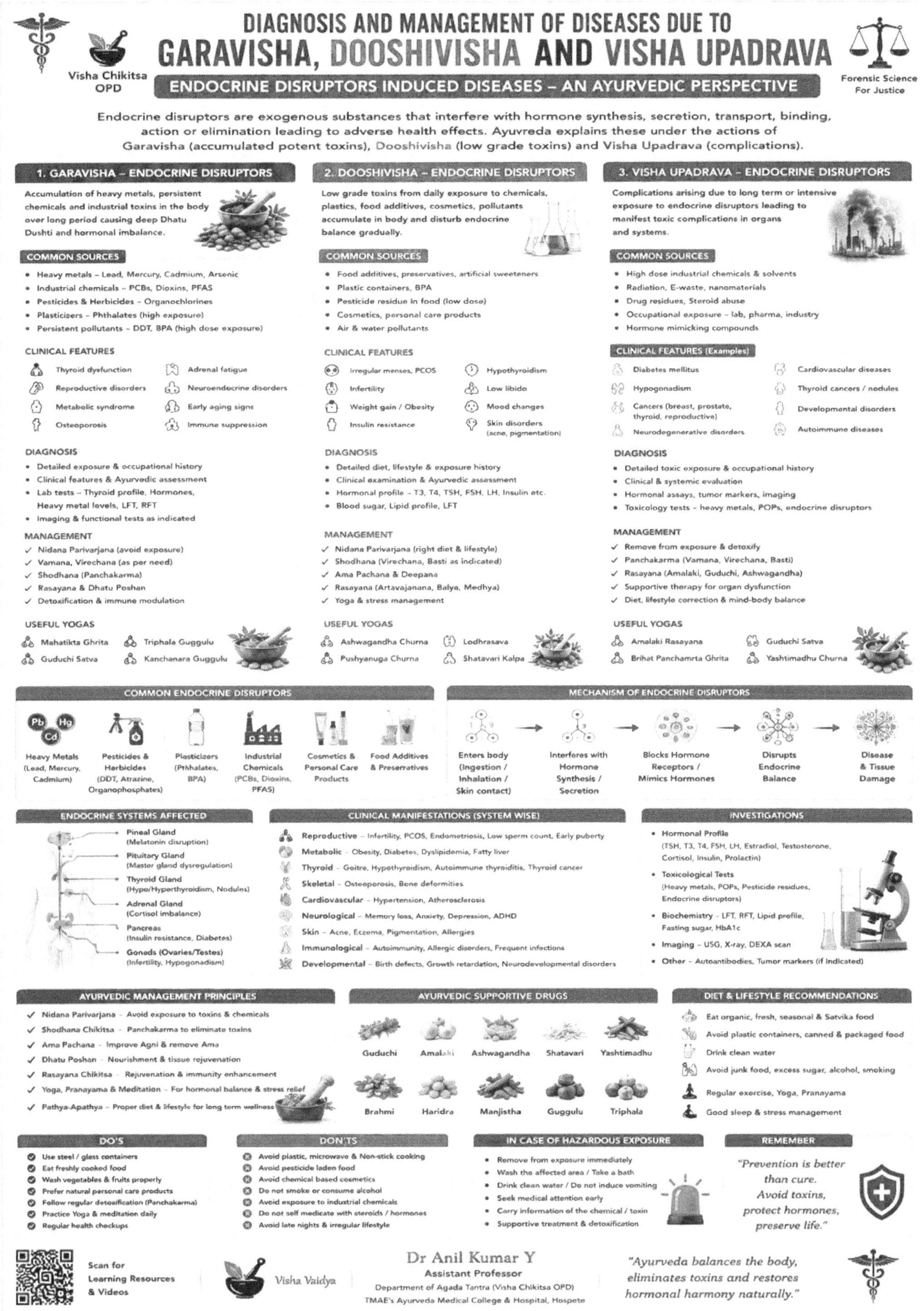
Visha Chikitsa OPD
DIAGNOSIS AND MANAGEMENT OF DISEASES DUE TO
GARAVISHA, DOOSHIVISHA AND VISHA UPADRAVA
ENDOCRINE DISRUPTORS INDUCED DISEASES – AN AYURVEDIC PERSPECTIVE
Forensic Science For Justice
Endocrine disruptors are exogenous substances that interfere with hormone synthesis, secretion, transport, binding, action or elimination leading to adverse health effects. Ayurveda explains these under the actions of Garavisha (accumulated potent toxins), Dooshivisha (low grade toxins) and Visha Upadrava (complications).
1. GARAVISHA – ENDOCRINE DISRUPTORS
Accumulation of heavy metals, persistent chemicals and industrial toxins in the body over long period causing deep Dhatu Dushti and hormonal imbalance.
COMMON SOURCES
• Heavy metals – Lead, Mercury, Cadmium, Arsenic
• Industrial chemicals – PCBs, Dioxins, PFAS
• Pesticides & Herbicides – Organochlorines
• Plasticizers – Phthalates (high exposure)
• Persistent pollutants – DDT, BPA (high dose exposure)
CLINICAL FEATURES
Thyroid dysfunction
Adrenal fatigue
Reproductive disorders
Neuroendocrine disorders
Metabolic syndrome
Early aging signs
Osteoporosis
Immune suppression
DIAGNOSIS
• Detailed exposure & occupational history
• Clinical features & Ayurvedic assessment
• Lab tests – Thyroid profile, Hormones, Heavy metal levels, LFT, RFT
• Imaging & functional tests as indicated
MANAGEMENT
✓ Nidana Parivarjana (avoid exposure)
✓ Vamana, Virechana (as per need)
✓ Shodhana (Panchakarma)
✓ Rasayana & Dhatu Poshan
✓ Detoxification & immune modulation
USEFUL YOGAS
Mahatikta Ghrita
Triphala Guggulu
Guduchi Satva
Kanchanara Guggulu
2. DOOSHIVISHA – ENDOCRINE DISRUPTORS
Low grade toxins from daily exposure to chemicals, plastics, food additives, cosmetics, pollutants accumulate in body and disturb endocrine balance gradually.
COMMON SOURCES
• Food additives, preservatives, artificial sweeteners
• Plastic containers, BPA
• Pesticide residue in food (low dose)
• Cosmetics, personal care products
• Air & water pollutants
CLINICAL FEATURES
Irregular menses, PCOS
Hypothyroidism
Infertility
Low libido
Weight gain / Obesity
Mood changes
Insulin resistance
Skin disorders (acne, pigmentation)
DIAGNOSIS
• Detailed diet, lifestyle & exposure history
• Clinical examination & Ayurvedic assessment
• Hormonal profile – T3, T4, TSH, FSH, LH, Insulin etc.
• Blood sugar, Lipid profile, LFT
MANAGEMENT
✓ Nidana Parivarjana (right diet & lifestyle)
✓ Shodhana (Virechana, Basti as indicated)
✓ Ama Pachana & Deepana
✓ Rasayana (Artavajanana, Balya, Medhya)
✓ Yoga & stress management
USEFUL YOGAS
Ashwagandha Churna
Lodhrasava
Pushyanuga Churna
Shatavari Kalpa
3. VISHA UPADRAVA – ENDOCRINE DISRUPTORS
Complications arising due to long term or intensive exposure to endocrine disruptors leading to manifest toxic complications in organs and systems.
COMMON SOURCES
• High dose industrial chemicals & solvents
• Radiation, E-waste, nanomaterials
• Drug residues, Steroid abuse
• Occupational exposure – lab, pharma, industry
• Hormone mimicking compounds
CLINICAL FEATURES (Examples)
Diabetes mellitus
Cardiovascular diseases
Hypogonadism
Thyroid cancers / nodules
Cancers (breast, prostate, thyroid, reproductive)
Developmental disorders
Neurodegenerative disorders
Autoimmune diseases
DIAGNOSIS
• Detailed toxic exposure & occupational history
• Clinical & systemic evaluation
• Hormonal assays, tumor markers, imaging
• Toxicology tests – heavy metals, POPs, endocrine disruptors
MANAGEMENT
✓ Remove from exposure & detoxify
✓ Panchakarma (Vamana, Virechana, Basti)
✓ Rasayana (Amalaki, Guduchi, Ashwagandha)
✓ Supportive therapy for organ dysfunction
✓ Diet, lifestyle correction & mind-body balance
USEFUL YOGAS
Amalaki Rasayana
Guduchi Satva
Brihat Panchamrta Ghrita
Yashtimadhu Churna
COMMON ENDOCRINE DISRUPTORS
Pb Hg Cd
Heavy Metals (Lead, Mercury, Cadmium)
Pesticides & Herbicides (DDT, Atrazine, Organophosphates)
Plasticizers (Phthalates, BPA)
Industrial Chemicals (PCBs, Dioxins, PFAS)
Cosmetics & Personal Care Products
Food Additives & Preservatives
MECHANISM OF ENDOCRINE DISRUPTORS
Enters body (Ingestion / Inhalation / Skin contact) → Interferes with Hormone Synthesis / Secretion → Blocks Hormone Receptors / Mimics Hormones → Disrupts Endocrine Balance → Disease & Tissue Damage
ENDOCRINE SYSTEMS AFFECTED
Pineal Gland (Melatonin disruption)
Pituitary Gland (Master gland dysregulation)
Thyroid Gland (Hypo/Hyperthyroidism, Nodules)
Adrenal Gland (Cortisol imbalance)
Pancreas (Insulin resistance, Diabetes)
Gonads (Ovaries/Testes) (Infertility, Hypogonadism)
CLINICAL MANIFESTATIONS (SYSTEM WISE)
Reproductive – Infertility, PCOS, Endometriosis, Low sperm count, Early puberty
Metabolic – Obesity, Diabetes, Dyslipidemia, Fatty liver
Thyroid – Goitre, Hypothyroidism, Autoimmune thyroiditis, Thyroid cancer
Skeletal – Osteoporosis, Bone deformities
Cardiovascular – Hypertension, Atherosclerosis
Neurological – Memory loss, Anxiety, Depression, ADHD
Skin – Acne, Eczema, Pigmentation, Allergies
Immunological – Autoimmunity, Allergic disorders, Frequent infections
Developmental – Birth defects, Growth retardation, Neurodevelopmental disorders
INVESTIGATIONS
• Hormonal Profile (TSH, T3, T4, FSH, LH, Estradiol, Testosterone, Cortisol, Insulin, Prolactin)
• Toxicological Tests (Heavy metals, POPs, Pesticide residues, Endocrine disruptors)
• Biochemistry – LFT, RFT, Lipid profile, Fasting sugar, HbA1c
• Imaging – USG, X-ray, DEXA scan
• Other – Autoantibodies, Tumor markers (if indicated)
AYURVEDIC MANAGEMENT PRINCIPLES
✓ Nidana Parivarjana – Avoid exposure to toxins & chemicals
✓ Shodhana Chikitsa – Panchakarma to eliminate toxins
✓ Ama Pachana – Improve Agni & remove Ama
✓ Dhatu Poshan – Nourishment & tissue rejuvenation
✓ Rasayana Chikitsa – Rejuvenation & immunity enhancement
✓ Yoga, Pranayama & Meditation – For hormonal balance & stress relief
✓ Pathya-Apathya – Proper diet & lifestyle for long term wellness
AYURVEDIC SUPPORTIVE DRUGS
Guduchi
Amalaki
Ashwagandha
Shatavari
Yashtimadhu
Brahmi
Haridra
Manjistha
Guggulu
Triphala
DIET & LIFESTYLE RECOMMENDATIONS
Eat organic, fresh, seasonal & Satvika food
Avoid plastic containers, canned & packaged food
Drink clean water
Avoid junk food, excess sugar, alcohol, smoking
Regular exercise, Yoga, Pranayama
Good sleep & stress management
DO'S
Use steel / glass containers
Eat freshly cooked food
Wash vegetables & fruits properly
Prefer natural personal care products
Follow regular detoxification (Panchakarma)
Practice Yoga & meditation daily
Regular health checkups
DON'TS
Avoid plastic, microwave & Non-stick cooking
Avoid pesticide laden food
Avoid chemical based cosmetics
Do not smoke or consume alcohol
Avoid exposure to industrial chemicals
Do not self medicate with steroids / hormones
Avoid late nights & irregular lifestyle
IN CASE OF HAZARDOUS EXPOSURE
• Remove from exposure immediately
• Wash the affected area / Take a bath
• Drink clean water / Do not induce vomiting
• Seek medical attention early
• Carry information of the chemical / toxin
• Supportive treatment & detoxification
REMEMBER
"Prevention is better than cure. Avoid toxins, protect hormones, preserve life."
Scan for Learning Resources & Videos
Visha Vaidya
Dr Anil Kumar Y
Assistant Professor
Department of Agada Tantra (Visha Chikitsa OPD)
TMAE's Ayurveda Medical College & Hospital, Hospete
"Ayurveda balances the body, eliminates toxins and restores hormonal harmony naturally."

PRACTICAL NO. 3

DOOSHIVISHA / GARAVISHA CASE RECORD

Endocrine Disruptors Induced Diseases

Case No:05

Date:

Patient Details

Name::

Age::

Sex:

Address:

Occupation:

Chief Complaints:

History of Present Illness:

Exposure History:

Nidana:

Examination:

Samprapti:

Differential Diagnosis:

Diagnosis:

Treatment Given

Outcome

Discussion

Faculty Signature

DIAGNOSIS & MANAGEMENT OF DERMATOLOGICAL MANIFESTATIONS DUE TO VISHA

Visha Chikitsa OPD

EXAMPLES: CONTACT POISONING (PADUKA VISHA, ABHARANA VISHA ETC.)

"Visha Sparsha Ja Vikarah Twakgate Rogarupinah" → *Charaka Chikitsa Sthana 23/5*

Contact poisoning occurs when the skin comes in direct contact with toxic substances (natural, metallic, chemical or plant origin) leading to local and systemic reactions.

1. COMMON EXAMPLES OF CONTACT POISONING (VISHA)

PADUKA VISHA (Footwear Poisoning)

Due to leather, synthetic material, dyes, adhesives, rubber chemicals.

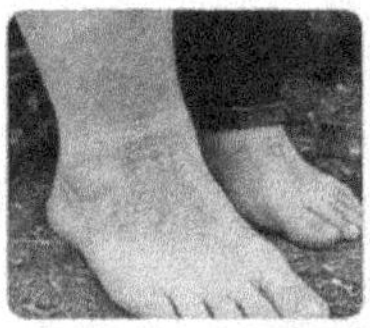

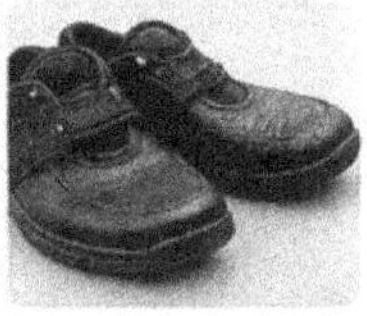

- Itching, redness, blisters
- Fissuring, burning sensation
- Chronic dermatitis

ABHARANA VISHA (Ornamental Metal Poisoning)

Due to nickel, cobalt, chromium, mercury, impure gold/silver alloys.

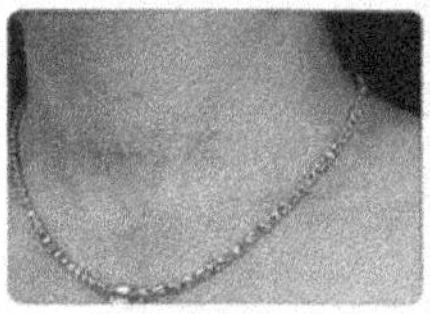

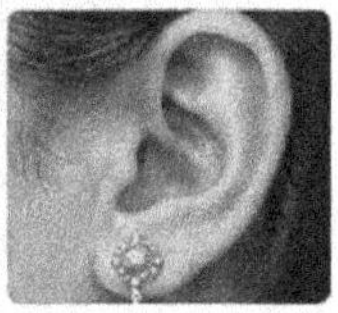

- Erythema, itching at contact site
- Papules, oozing, discoloration
- Eczematous or lichenoid eruptions

OTHER CONTACT VISHA

Plants (Lantana, Poison ivy), Chemicals (acids, alkalis, detergents, pesticides, cosmetics etc.)

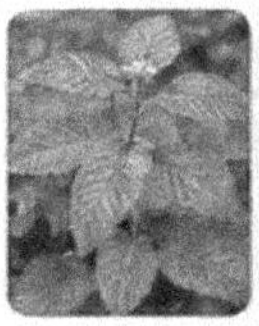

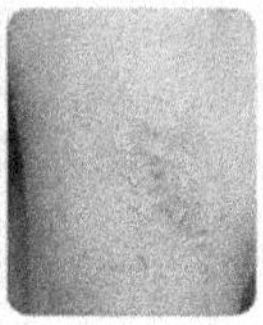

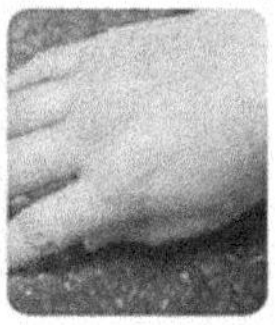

- Redness, burning, itching
- Vesicles, bullae, pigmentation
- May lead to ulceration in severe cases

2. CLINICAL PRESENTATIONS

TYPE OF REACTION	LOCAL FEATURES	SYSTEMIC FEATURES	POSSIBLE CAUSE	CLINICAL IMAGES (EXAMPLES)
Mild (Irritant Contact Dermatitis)	Redness, itching, mild burning, dryness	Usually absent	Detergents, soaps, rubber, leather	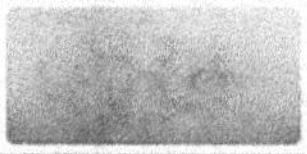 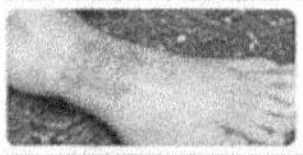
Moderate (Allergic Contact Dermatitis)	Erythema, papules, vesicles, oozing, itching	Sometimes – malaise, headache	Nickel, cosmetic chemicals, dyes	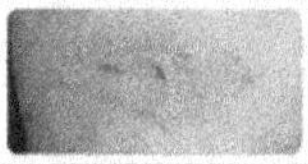 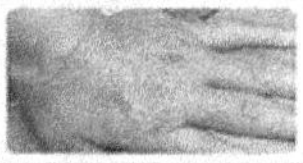
Severe (Toxic Contact Dermatitis)	Blisters, bullae, ulceration, cracking, severe pain	Fever, giddiness, nausea, weakness, rarely shock	Acids, alkalis, pesticides, mercury, arsenic, strong chemicals	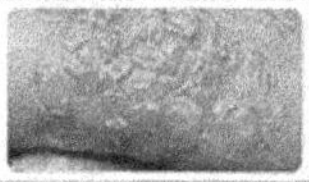 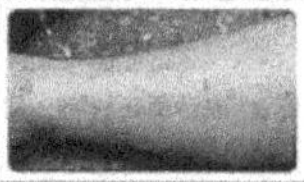

3. DIAGNOSIS

- ☑ Detailed history: nature of contact, duration, site, timing of onset.
- ☑ Inspection of lesions: erythema, vesicles, bullae, pigmentation, lichenification.
- ☑ Patch test (in suspected allergic cases).
- ☑ Rule out infections or other dermatological disorders.
- ☑ Laboratory (if needed): CBC, LFT, RFT, serum IgE (in severe/allergic cases).

KEY POINTS

Early recognition prevents complications and chronic skin disorders.

4. MANAGEMENT (VISHA CHIKITSA APPROACH)

A. GENERAL MANAGEMENT

- ☑ Remove the source of contact.
- ☑ Clean the affected area with lukewarm water.
- ☑ Avoid scratching.
- ☑ Wear protective clothing/gloves.
- ☑ Supportive care – rest, hydration.

B. AYURVEDA MANAGEMENT

SHODHANA (If indicated)

- Virechana (Purgation)
- Raktamokshana (Bloodletting)

SHAMANA CHIKITSA

- Internal Medicines:
  - Gandhaka Rasayana
  - Khadira Guggulu
  - Mahamanjishtadi Kashaya
  - Arogyavardhini Vati
  - Panchtikta Ghrita Guggulu
- External Applications:
  - Lepa: Chandana, Yashtimadhu, Haridra, Nimba
  - Prakshalana: Triphala Kashaya, Nimba Kwatha
  - Takradhara / Parisheka

5. MODERN MANAGEMENT (AS PER SEVERITY)

SEVERITY	TREATMENT
Mild	Antihistamines (e.g., Cetirizine), Topical calamine, emollients
Moderate	Topical corticosteroids, oral antihistamines, Barrier creams
Severe	Systemic steroids (if needed), antibiotics (if infected), IV fluids (if toxic)

PREVENTION

- Use hypoallergenic footwear & ornaments
- Avoid direct contact with chemicals & toxins
- Wear gloves, protective clothing
- Clean skin properly after exposure
- Use herbal cosmetics whenever possible

WHEN TO REFER?

- Extensive skin involvement
- Systemic symptoms
- Suspected toxic exposure
- No improvement with initial care

Dr Anil Kumar Y
Assistant professor
Department of Agadatantra

RECOGNIZE EARLY • TREAT WISELY • PREVENT EXPOSURE • PROTECT SKIN HEALTH

PRACTICAL NO. 4

DERMATOLOGICAL MANIFESTATIONS OF VISHA

Contact Poisoning(ABHARANA)

Case No:01

Date:

Patient Details

Name::

Age::

Sex:

Address:

Occupation:

Chief Complaints:

History of Present Illness:

Exposure History:

Nidana:

Examination:

Samprapti:

Differential Diagnosis:

Diagnosis:

Treatment Given

Outcome

Discussion

Faculty Signature

PRACTICAL NO. 4

DERMATOLOGICAL MANIFESTATIONS OF VISHA

Contact Poisoning (ALLERGIC DERMATITIS)

Case No:02

Date:

Patient Details

Name::

Age::

Sex:

Address:

Occupation:

Chief Complaints:

History of Present Illness:

Exposure History:

Nidana:

Examination:

Samprapti:

Differential Diagnosis:

Diagnosis:

Treatment Given

Outcome

Discussion

Faculty Signature

PRACTICAL NO. 4

DERMATOLOGICAL MANIFESTATIONS OF VISHA

Contact Poisoning (IRRITANT DERMATITIS)

Case No:03

Date:

Patient Details

Name::

Age::

Sex:

Address:

Occupation:

Chief Complaints:

History of Present Illness:

Exposure History:

Nidana:

Examination:

Samprapti:

Differential Diagnosis:

Diagnosis:

Treatment Given

Outcome

Discussion

Faculty Signature

DIAGNOSIS AND MANAGEMENT OF DERMATOLOGICAL MANIFESTATIONS DUE TO VISHA – BITES AND STINGS

Visha Chikitsa OPD

EARLY RECOGNITION • ACCURATE DIAGNOSIS • PROMPT MANAGEMENT • SAVE LIVES

Bites and stings from poisonous creatures can cause local skin reactions and systemic toxicity. Timely identification, appropriate diagnosis and proper management prevent complications.

1. COMMON BITES & STINGS CAUSING DERMATOLOGICAL MANIFESTATIONS

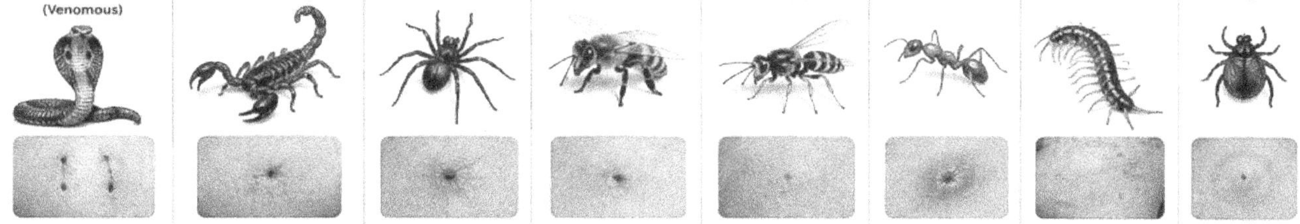

SNAKE BITE (Venomous)	SCORPION STING	SPIDER BITE	BEE STING	WASP STING	ANT BITE	CENTIPEDE BITE	TICK BITE
• Puncture marks (1 or 2) • Local pain, swelling, bruising, blister • May progress to necrosis	• Local severe pain, • redness, swelling • Paresthesia, sweating	• Redness, pain, itching • May form blisters or necrosis	• Immediate sharp pain • Redness, swelling, urticaria • May cause anaphylaxis	• Painful sting • Erythema, swelling, urticaria	• Burning pain • Pustule formation • Itching	• Severe pain • Redness, swelling, vesicles	• Itching, redness • May transmit infections

2. CLINICAL PRESENTATIONS

BITE / STING	LOCAL FEATURES	SYSTEMIC FEATURES	POSSIBLE COMPLICATIONS
SNAKE BITE	• Pain, swelling, erythema • Blister, ecchymosis • Necrosis (in severe cases)	• Nausea, vomiting • Ptosis, diplopia • Respiratory distress • Bleeding manifestations	• Tissue necrosis • Compartment syndrome • Renal failure, shock
SCORPION STING	• Intense pain, erythema • Burning sensation	• Profuse sweating • Salivation, vomiting • Hypertension / Hypotension • Tachycardia, arrhythmia	• Pulmonary edema • Cardiac failure • Shock
SPIDER BITE	• Redness, pain, swelling • Blister /necrosis (some species)	• Fever, malaise • Myalgia, restlessness	• Necrotic ulcer • Secondary infection
BEE / WASP STING	• Pain, redness, swelling • Urticaria	• Generalized urticaria • Bronchospasm • Anaphylactic shock	• Anaphylaxis • Airway obstruction
ANT BITE	• Burning pain • Pustule / vesicle formation	• Itching • Mild fever (rare)	• Secondary infection • Allergic reaction
CENTIPEDE BITE	• Severe pain, redness • Swelling, vesicles	• Nausea, vomiting • Restlessness, giddiness	• Hypotension • Respiratory distress (rare)
TICK BITE	• Erythema, itching • Local inflammation	• Fever, headache • Malaise, rash (Lyme disease)	• Lyme disease • Tick paralysis (rare)

3. DIAGNOSTIC APPROACH

- ☑ **Detailed history:** Time, place, activity, type of creature.
- ☑ **Examination:** Site, number of puncture marks, local reactions.
- ☑ **Identification of creature** (if possible).
- ☑ Look for systemic symptoms.
- ☑ **Investigations** (if needed):
  - CBC, ESR, CRP
  - Coagulation profile
  - Renal function tests
  - Serum electrolytes
  - X-ray / USG (in complications)
- ☑ Rule out secondary infections.

4. MANAGEMENT APPROACH

A. GENERAL PRINCIPLES (ALL BITES & STINGS)

1. Reassure patient and keep calm.
2. Immobilize the affected part.
3. Remove rings, watches, tight clothing.
4. Clean the area with soap and water.
5. Avoid cutting, sucking or applying irritants.
6. Monitor vitals and watch for systemic signs.

Key: Early management prevents severe complications.

B. MODERN MANAGEMENT

Pain & Inflammation	Analgesics (Paracetamol / NSAIDs), Ice pack (if swelling)
Allergic Reactions	Antihistamines (Cetirizine, Levocetirizine), Topical / Oral steroids (as needed)
Severe Allergy / Anaphylaxis	Adrenaline (IM), Oxygen, IV fluids, Steroids, Antihistamines
Infection	Topical antibiotics, Oral antibiotics (if infected)
Tetanus Prophylaxis	Tetanus toxoid as per status
Specific Management	Snake bite → ASV (as per indication) Scorpion sting → Prazosin (if needed) Tick bite → Doxycycline (if Lyme suspected)

C. AYURVEDA MANAGEMENT (VISHA CHIKITSA)

SHODHANA (If indicated)
- Vamana (in suitable cases)
- Virechana
- Rakta Mokshana (Alabu, Jalauka)

SHAMANA CHIKITSA

Internal Medicines:
- Gandhaka Rasayana
- Mahamrityunjaya Rasa
- Kaishora Guggulu
- Arogyavardhini Vati
- Panchatikta Ghrita Guggulu

External Applications:
- **Lepa:** Chandana, Yashtimadhu, Haridra, Nimba, Jatamansi
- **Prakshalana:** Triphala Kashaya, Nimba Kashaya
- **Taila:** Jatyadi Taila, Nimba Taila

5. FIRST AID – DOS & DON'TS

DO'S	DON'TS
✓ Keep the patient calm	✗ Do not cut or incise
✓ Clean the bite/sting site	✗ Do not suck venom
✓ Apply cold compress	✗ Do not apply chemicals, mud, or irritants
✓ Immobilize the part	✗ Do not give alcohol
✓ Seek medical help early	✗ Do not delay treatment

6. PREVENTION

- Wear protective clothing & footwear
- Avoid sleeping on the floor
- Keep surroundings clean
- Insect repellents
- Avoid touching unknown creatures

7. WHEN TO REFER IMMEDIATELY?

- Difficulty in breathing
- Persistent vomiting
- Profuse sweating / salivation
- Confusion / restlessness
- Bleeding manifestations
- Swelling spreading rapidly
- Signs of shock

Dr Anil Kumar Y
Assistant professor
Department of Agadatantra

Visha Vaidya

IDENTIFY EARLY • TREAT PROMPTLY • PREVENT COMPLICATIONS • SAVE LIVES

DERMATOLOGICAL MANIFESTATIONS OF VISHA BITES (DOG BITE)

Visha Chikitsa OPD

Forensic Science For Justice

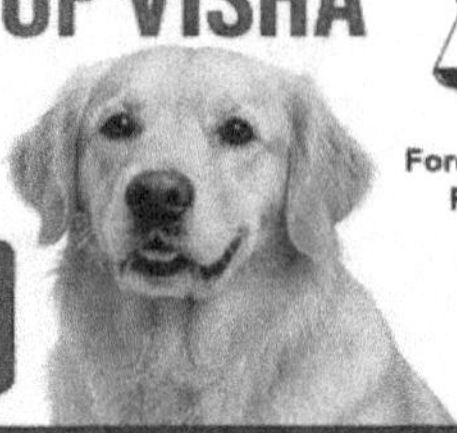

Dog bite is a Visha (toxic) trauma that can lead to local tissue injury and systemic complications. Early recognition of dermatological manifestations is crucial for prompt management and prevention of infections and rabies.

1. CLINICAL PRESENTATIONS – DERMATOLOGICAL MANIFESTATIONS

A. IMMEDIATE (0–6 HOURS)
- Puncture wounds
- Scratch marks
- Bleeding
- Pain & tenderness
- Local redness

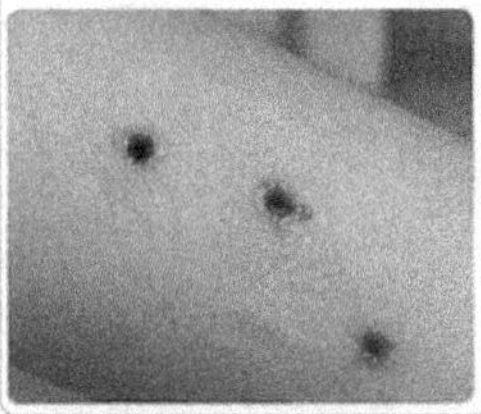

B. EARLY (6–72 HOURS)
- Redness & swelling
- Warmth
- Pain & itching
- Multiple bite marks
- Oozing / serous discharge

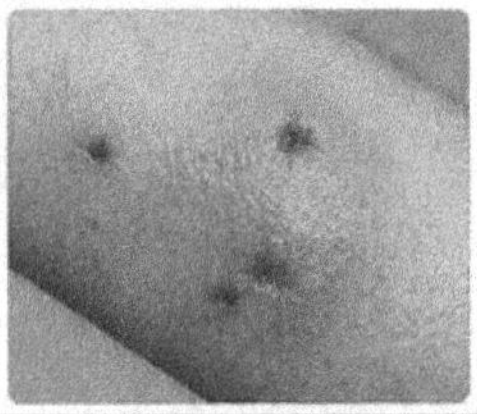

C. ESTABLISHED INFECTION (3–7 DAYS)
- Increased redness
- Swelling
- Pus discharge
- Induration
- Crusting / scab formation

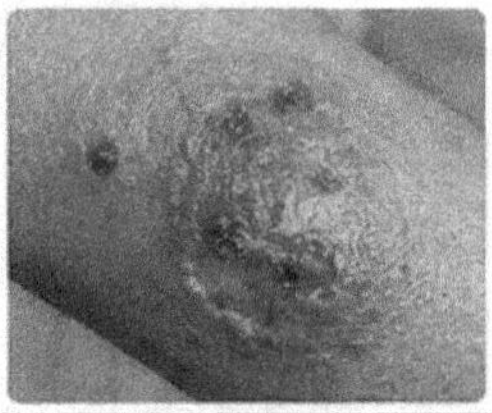

D. ADVANCED / COMPLICATIONS (> 7 DAYS)
- Abscess formation
- Cellulitis
- Lymphangitis
- Ulceration
- Necrosis (rare)

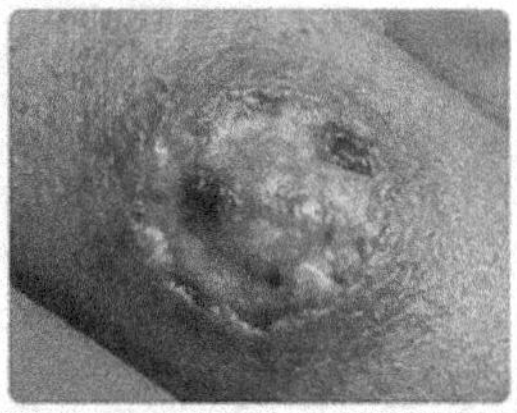

E. HEALING STAGE (AFTER TREATMENT)
- Gradual reduction of redness
- Scab fall
- Granulation tissue
- Scar formation

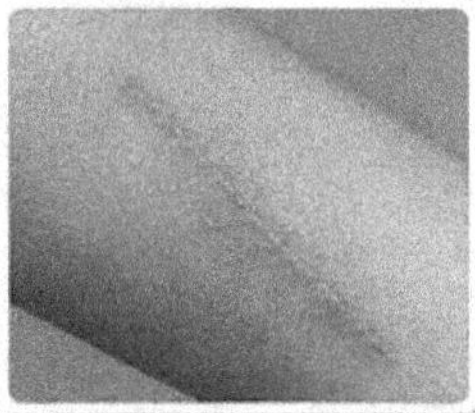

2. TYPES OF DOG BITE WOUNDS

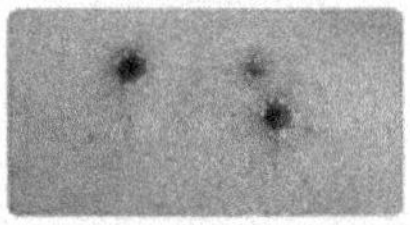

PUNCTURE WOUND
Deep, narrow, caused by canine teeth.
High risk of infection & tetanus.

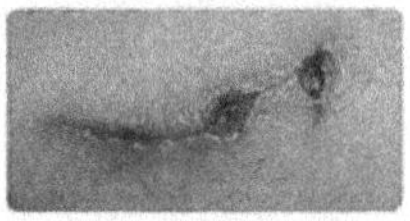

LACERATED WOUND
Irregular tear of skin and underlying tissue.
May bleed profusely.

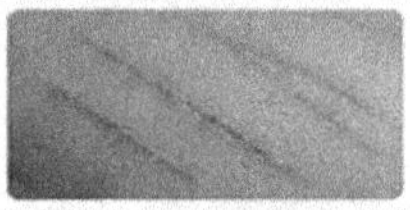

ABRASION / SCRATCH
Superficial skin injury caused by claw or rough contact.

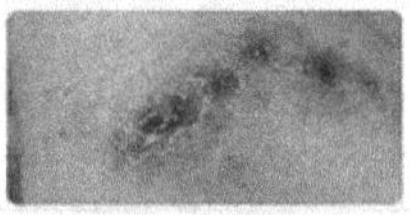

CRUSH INJURY
Tissue damage due to strong bite force.
May cause devitalized tissue.

3. SIGNS OF LOCAL INFECTION

- Redness
- Swelling
- Warmth
- Pain & tenderness
- Pus discharge
- Fever (systemic sign)

4. COMPLICATIONS

- Cellulitis
- Abscess
- Lymphangitis
- Septicemia
- Tetanus
- Rabies (Neurotropic virus)

5. DIFFERENTIAL DIAGNOSIS

- Insect bite
- Cat bite
- Human bite
- Spider bite
- Pyoderma
- Necrotizing fasciitis
- Allergic contact dermatitis

6. CLINICAL PEARLS

- ✓ Dog bites are polymicrobial.
- ✓ Deeper puncture wounds are more prone to infection.
- ✓ Observe for signs of rabies in the animal.
- ✓ Post-exposure prophylaxis (anti-rabies vaccine ± RIG) is essential.
- ✓ Tetanus prophylaxis must not be missed.

7. MANAGEMENT

A. IMMEDIATE WOUND CARE
- Wash the wound under running water with soap for 15 minutes
- Remove dirt & devitalized tissue
- Apply povidone iodine solution
- Avoid primary suturing (unless essential)

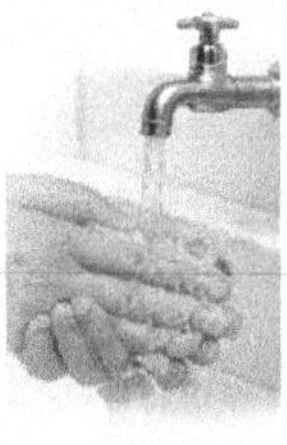

B. MEDICAL MANAGEMENT
- Antibiotics (Amoxicillin-Clavulanate / Doxycycline + Metronidazole)
- Analgesics for pain relief
- Anti-inflammatory drugs
- Anti-rabies vaccination (as per WHO schedule)
- Rabies Immunoglobulin (in severe exposures)
- Tetanus toxoid / TT booster

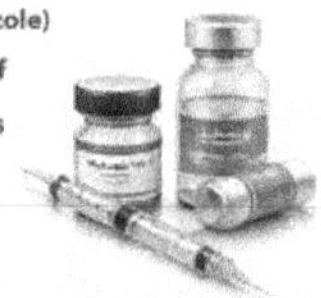

C. AYURVEDIC SUPPORTIVE CARE (Visha Chikitsa)
- Vranashodhana – cleansing with Panchavalkala Kwatha
- Vranaropana – Jatyadi Taila / Yashada Bhasma
- Gandhaka Rasayana / Haridra Khanda
- Aarogya Vardhaka – Guduchi, Nimba, Amalaki
- Pathya – Laghu, Satvika Ahara
- Avoid Viruddha Ahara & Nidravana (excessive sleep)

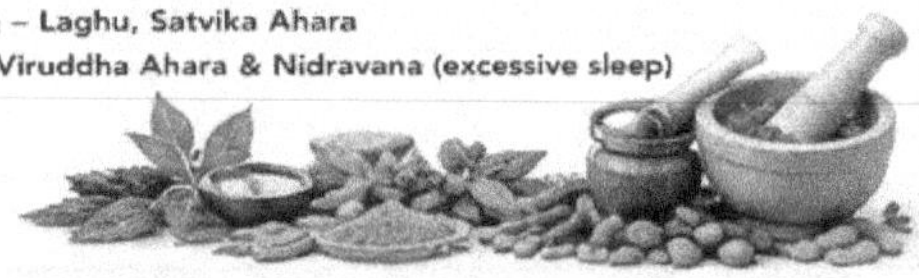

8. RABIES – WARNING SIGNS (IN ANIMAL)

- Change in behaviour (aggression / restlessness)
- Excess salivation
- Difficulty in swallowing
- Paralysis
- Death

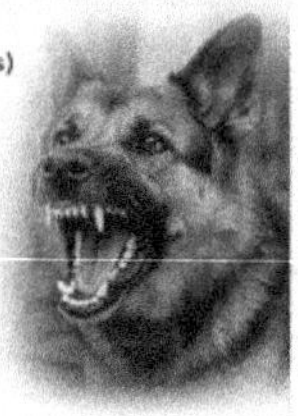

9. WHEN TO REFER

- Deep wounds / gaping injuries
- Neurovascular damage
- Signs of systemic infection
- Immunocompromised patients
- Delayed presentation (>24 hrs)
- Suspected rabies exposure

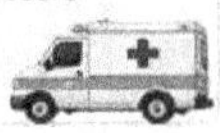

10. PREVENTION

- Avoid teasing or provoking dogs
- Do not feed unfamiliar dogs
- Vaccinate pet dogs regularly
- Report stray dog menace
- Awareness about animal behaviour and rabies

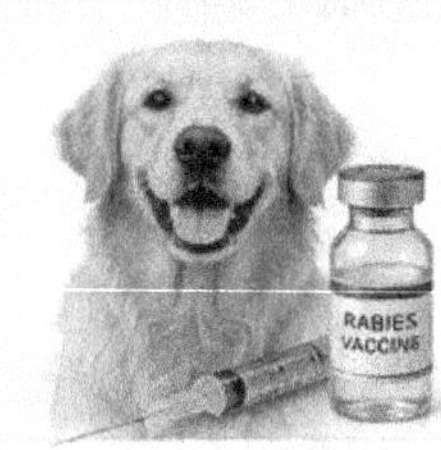

Visha Vaidya

Dr Anil Kumar Y
Assistant Professor
Department of Agada Tantra (Visha Chikitsa OPD)
TMAE'S Ayurveda Medical College & Hospital, Hospete

"Early care of a dog bite prevents infection and protects life."

PRACTICAL NO. 4

DERMATOLOGICAL MANIFESTATIONS OF VISHA

BITES(DOG Bite)

Case No:04

Date:

Patient Details

Name::

Age::

Sex:

Address:

Occupation:

Chief Complaints:

History of Present Illness:

Exposure History:

Nidana:

Examination:

Samprapti:

Differential Diagnosis:

Diagnosis:

Treatment Given

Outcome

Discussion

Faculty Signature

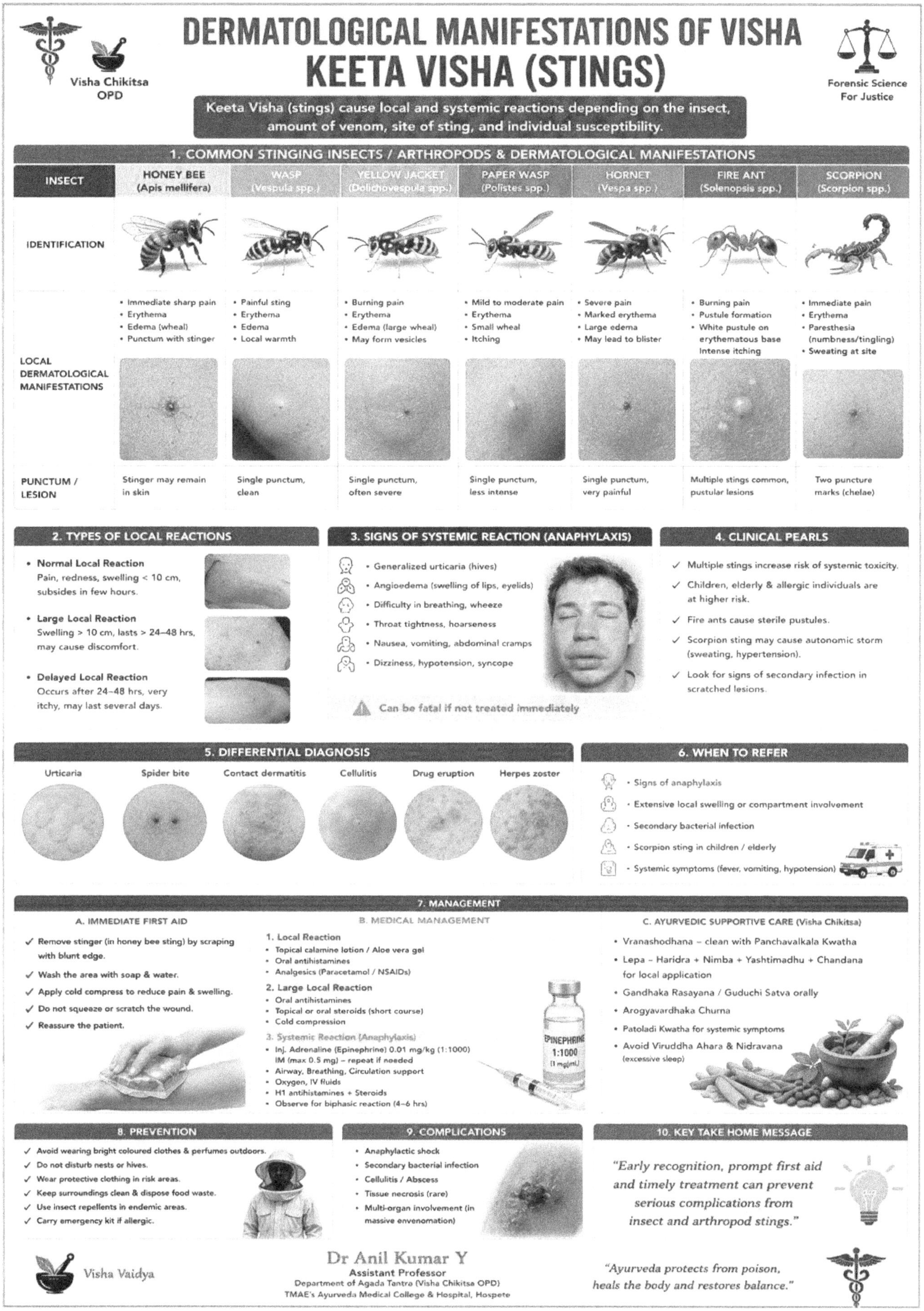
Visha Chikitsa OPD
DERMATOLOGICAL MANIFESTATIONS OF VISHA
KEETA VISHA (STINGS)
Forensic Science For Justice
Keeta Visha (stings) cause local and systemic reactions depending on the insect, amount of venom, site of sting, and individual susceptibility.
1. COMMON STINGING INSECTS / ARTHROPODS & DERMATOLOGICAL MANIFESTATIONS
INSECT
HONEY BEE (Apis mellifera)
WASP (Vespula spp.)
YELLOW JACKET (Dolichovespula spp.)
PAPER WASP (Polistes spp.)
HORNET (Vespa spp.)
FIRE ANT (Solenopsis spp.)
SCORPION (Scorpion spp.)
IDENTIFICATION
LOCAL DERMATOLOGICAL MANIFESTATIONS
• Immediate sharp pain • Erythema • Edema (wheal) • Puncture with stinger
• Painful sting • Erythema • Edema • Local warmth
• Burning pain • Erythema • Edema (large wheal) • May form vesicles
• Mild to moderate pain • Erythema • Small wheal • Itching
• Severe pain • Marked erythema • Large edema • May lead to blister
• Burning pain • Pustule formation • White pustule on erythematous base Intense itching
• Immediate pain • Erythema • Paresthesia (numbness/tingling) • Sweating at site
PUNCTUM / LESION
Stinger may remain in skin
Single punctum, clean
Single punctum, often severe
Single punctum, less intense
Single punctum, very painful
Multiple stings common, pustular lesions
Two puncture marks (chelae)
2. TYPES OF LOCAL REACTIONS
• Normal Local Reaction
Pain, redness, swelling < 10 cm, subsides in few hours.
• Large Local Reaction
Swelling > 10 cm, lasts > 24–48 hrs, may cause discomfort.
• Delayed Local Reaction
Occurs after 24–48 hrs, very itchy, may last several days.
3. SIGNS OF SYSTEMIC REACTION (ANAPHYLAXIS)
• Generalized urticaria (hives)
• Angioedema (swelling of lips, eyelids)
• Difficulty in breathing, wheeze
• Throat tightness, hoarseness
• Nausea, vomiting, abdominal cramps
• Dizziness, hypotension, syncope
Can be fatal if not treated immediately
4. CLINICAL PEARLS
✓ Multiple stings increase risk of systemic toxicity.
✓ Children, elderly & allergic individuals are at higher risk.
✓ Fire ants cause sterile pustules.
✓ Scorpion sting may cause autonomic storm (sweating, hypertension).
✓ Look for signs of secondary infection in scratched lesions.
5. DIFFERENTIAL DIAGNOSIS
Urticaria
Spider bite
Contact dermatitis
Cellulitis
Drug eruption
Herpes zoster
6. WHEN TO REFER
• Signs of anaphylaxis
• Extensive local swelling or compartment involvement
• Secondary bacterial infection
• Scorpion sting in children / elderly
• Systemic symptoms (fever, vomiting, hypotension)
7. MANAGEMENT
A. IMMEDIATE FIRST AID
✓ Remove stinger (in honey bee sting) by scraping with blunt edge.
✓ Wash the area with soap & water.
✓ Apply cold compress to reduce pain & swelling.
✓ Do not squeeze or scratch the wound.
✓ Reassure the patient.
B. MEDICAL MANAGEMENT
1. Local Reaction
• Topical calamine lotion / Aloe vera gel
• Oral antihistamines
• Analgesics (Paracetamol / NSAIDs)
2. Large Local Reaction
• Oral antihistamines
• Topical or oral steroids (short course)
• Cold compression
3. Systemic Reaction (Anaphylaxis)
• Inj. Adrenaline (Epinephrine) 0.01 mg/kg (1:1000) IM (max 0.5 mg) – repeat if needed
• Airway, Breathing, Circulation support
• Oxygen, IV fluids
• H1 antihistamines + Steroids
• Observe for biphasic reaction (4–6 hrs)
EPINEPHRINE 1:1000 (1 mg/mL)
C. AYURVEDIC SUPPORTIVE CARE (Visha Chikitsa)
• Vranashodhana – clean with Panchavalkala Kwatha
• Lepa – Haridra + Nimba + Yashtimadhu + Chandana for local application
• Gandhaka Rasayana / Guduchi Satva orally
• Arogyavardhaka Churna
• Patoladi Kwatha for systemic symptoms
• Avoid Viruddha Ahara & Nidravana (excessive sleep)
8. PREVENTION
✓ Avoid wearing bright coloured clothes & perfumes outdoors.
✓ Do not disturb nests or hives.
✓ Wear protective clothing in risk areas.
✓ Keep surroundings clean & dispose food waste.
✓ Use insect repellents in endemic areas.
✓ Carry emergency kit if allergic.
9. COMPLICATIONS
• Anaphylactic shock
• Secondary bacterial infection
• Cellulitis / Abscess
• Tissue necrosis (rare)
• Multi-organ involvement (in massive envenomation)
10. KEY TAKE HOME MESSAGE
"Early recognition, prompt first aid and timely treatment can prevent serious complications from insect and arthropod stings."
Visha Vaidya
Dr Anil Kumar Y
Assistant Professor
Department of Agada Tantra (Visha Chikitsa OPD)
TMAE's Ayurveda Medical College & Hospital, Hospete
"Ayurveda protects from poison, heals the body and restores balance."

PRACTICAL NO. 4

DERMATOLOGICAL MANIFESTATIONS OF VISHA

KEETA VISHA(STINGS)

Case No:05

Date:

Patient Details

Name::

Age::

Sex:

Address:

Occupation:

Chief Complaints:

History of Present Illness:

Exposure History:

Nidana:

Examination:

Samprapti:

Differential Diagnosis:

Diagnosis:

Treatment Given

Outcome

Discussion

Faculty Signature

DIAGNOSIS & MANAGEMENT OF
CONTACT DERMATITIS
BASED ON THE PRINCIPLES OF
AGADA TANTRA & AGADA YOGAS

Visha Chikitsa OPD

"Visha Sparsha Ja Vikarah Twakgate Rogarupinah" – *Charaka Chikitsa Sthana 23/5*

Contact dermatitis is a *Twak Vikara* caused by the contact of skin with Visha (toxic substances) resulting in **Kandu (itching), Daha (burning), Raga (redness), Srava (oozing) and Pidaka (eruptions).**

1. CAUSES (VISHAS)

- Paduka Visha – Footwear materials, rubber, dyes, adhesives
- Abharana Visha – Ornaments made of nickel, cobalt, mercury, impure metals
- Varnashala Visha – Paints, chemicals, dyes, solvents
- Vanaspati Visha – Poison ivy, lantana, euphorbia, etc.
- Griha Visha – Detergents, soaps, cosmetics, acids, alkalis
- Krimija Visha – Insect bites, stings

2. SAMPRAPTI (Pathogenesis)

Visha Sparsha (Contact) → Tvak, Rakta, Mamsa Dushti → Pitta-Kapha Prakopa → Srotorodha → Utpatti of Kandu, Daha, Raga, Pidaka, Srava

DOSHA INVOLVEMENT

- **PITTA**: Daha, Raga, Pidaka, Srava
- **KAPHA**: Kandu, Picchila Srava, Shopha
- **RAKTA**: Raga, Daha, Pidaka

3. CLINICAL PRESENTATIONS

- Kandu (itching)
- Daha (burning sensation)
- Raga (erythema)
- Pidaka (papules / vesicles)
- Srava (oozing)
- Shyava / Vaivarnya (discoloration)
- Tvak Ruja (pain in severe cases)
- Shopha (swelling)

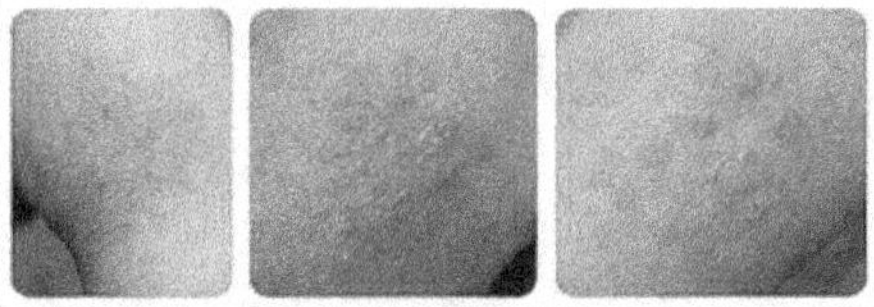

4. DIAGNOSIS (BASED ON AGADA TANTRA PRINCIPLES)

Detailed history:
- Nature of contact, duration, site, time of onset, previous exposure.

Observation of symptoms:
- Kandu, Daha, Pidaka, Srava, Raga, Shopha, Vaivarnya.

Pariksha (Examination):
- Nidan Parivarjana (identifying and removing the cause)
- Dosha involvement – mainly Pitta-Kapha with Rakta Dushti.

Differential diagnosis:
- Allergic dermatitis, urticaria, psoriasis, fungal infections.

5. CHIKITSA SUTRA (Line of Treatment)

"Nidana Parivarjana, Visha Shamana, Dosha Prashamana, Raktashodhana, Twak Prasadana."

Treatment principles:
- ☑ Remove the cause (Nidana Parivarjana)
- ☑ Shodhana (if required)
- ☑ Shamana (pacifying Doshas)
- ☑ Raktashodhana (purification of blood)
- ☑ Twak Prasadana (skin rejuvenation)

6. MANAGEMENT – AGADA TANTRA APPROACH

A. NIDANA PARIVARJANA
- Identify and completely avoid the causative Visha.

B. SHODHANA (If severe / chronic cases)
- Virechana – for Pitta-Kapha dominant cases
- Raktamokshana – in Rakta Dushti with severe symptoms
- Lepa with Tikta Dravyas before Shodhana

C. SHAMANA CHIKITSA
- Internal medicines (Visha Shamana, Raktaprasadana, Kandughna, Pittashamana)
- External applications (Lepa, Prakshalana, Parisheka)

D. TWAK PRASADANA
- Skin nourishment and regeneration with Rasayana and Varnya dravyas.

7. AGADA YOGAS (INTERNAL MEDICINES)

AGADA YOGA	MAIN INGREDIENTS	ACTION
Panchatikta Ghrita Guggulu	Tikta dravyas, Ghrita, Guggulu	Visha Shamana, Raktashodhana, Twak Vikara Nashana
Kaishora Guggulu	Guggulu, Triphala, Trikatu, Tikta dravyas	Raktashodhaka, Kandughna, Shothahara
Mahamanjishthadi Kwatha	Manjistha, Sariva, Nimba, Guduchi, Triphala	Raktaprasadana, Varnya, Pittashamana
Guduchi Satva	Guduchi	Visha Shamana, Immunomodulator
Sudarshana Churna	Tikta, Katu dravyas	Jwaraghna, Amapachana, VishaShamana

8. EXTERNAL APPLICATIONS (LEPA & OTHERS)

APPLICATION	DRUGS / DRAVYAS	INDICATIONS
Lepa (Paste)	Nimba Patra, Haridra, Lodhra, Yashtimadhu, Chandana	Kandu, Daha, Pidaka, Raga, Srava
Prakshalana (Wash)	Triphala Kwatha, Nimba Kwatha, Manjistha Kwatha	Itching, oozing, redness
Parisheka (Pouring)	Chandana, Ushira, Lodhra, Yashtimadhu Kwatha	Daha, burning, irritation
Taila / Ghrita	Nimba Taila, Mahatikta Ghrita	Dry, chronic, scaling dermatitis

9. MODERN CORRELATION

- Contact dermatitis is an inflammatory skin reaction due to irritant or allergic contact.
- **Pathophysiology:**
- Chemical penetrates → Skin barrier damage → Immune response → Inflammation.
- Symptoms: Erythema, vesicles, itching, edema, scaling.

10. DIET & PATHYA-APATHYA

PATHYA (To be followed)	APATHYA (To be avoided)
✔ Tikta, Katu, Kashaya Rasa	✗ Amla, Lavana, Katu excess
✔ Yava, Godhuma, Shali	✗ Curd, Fish, Alcohol
✔ Neem, Guduchi, Patola	✗ Day sleep
✔ Ghee in moderation	✗ Stress and anger
✔ Plenty of water	✗ Exposure to chemicals, dyes, heat
✔ Avoid heat exposure	

11. PREVENTION

- Avoid contact with known allergens
- Use protective gloves, footwear
- Use natural, non-toxic products
- Maintain skin hygiene
- Early treatment prevents chronicity

"Early recognition, removal of cause and Agada Chikitsa bring quick relief and prevent recurrence.

Dr Anil Kumar Y
Assistant professor
Department of Agadatantra

Visha Vaidya

PRACTICAL NO. 4

DERMATOLOGICAL MANIFESTATIONS OF VISHA

CONTACT DERMATITIS (STHAVARA VISHA)

Case No:06

Date:

Patient Details

Name::

Age::

Sex:

Address:

Occupation:

Chief Complaints:

History of Present Illness:

Exposure History:

Nidana:

Examination:

Samprapti:

Differential Diagnosis:

Diagnosis:

Treatment Given

Outcome

Discussion

Faculty Signature

PRACTICAL NO. 4

DERMATOLOGICAL MANIFESTATIONS OF VISHA

BITES/STINGS

Case No:07

Date:

Patient Details

Name::

Age::

Sex:

Address:

Occupation:

Chief Complaints:

History of Present Illness:

Exposure History:

Nidana:

Examination:

Samprapti:

Differential Diagnosis:

Diagnosis:

Treatment Given

Outcome

Discussion

Faculty Signature

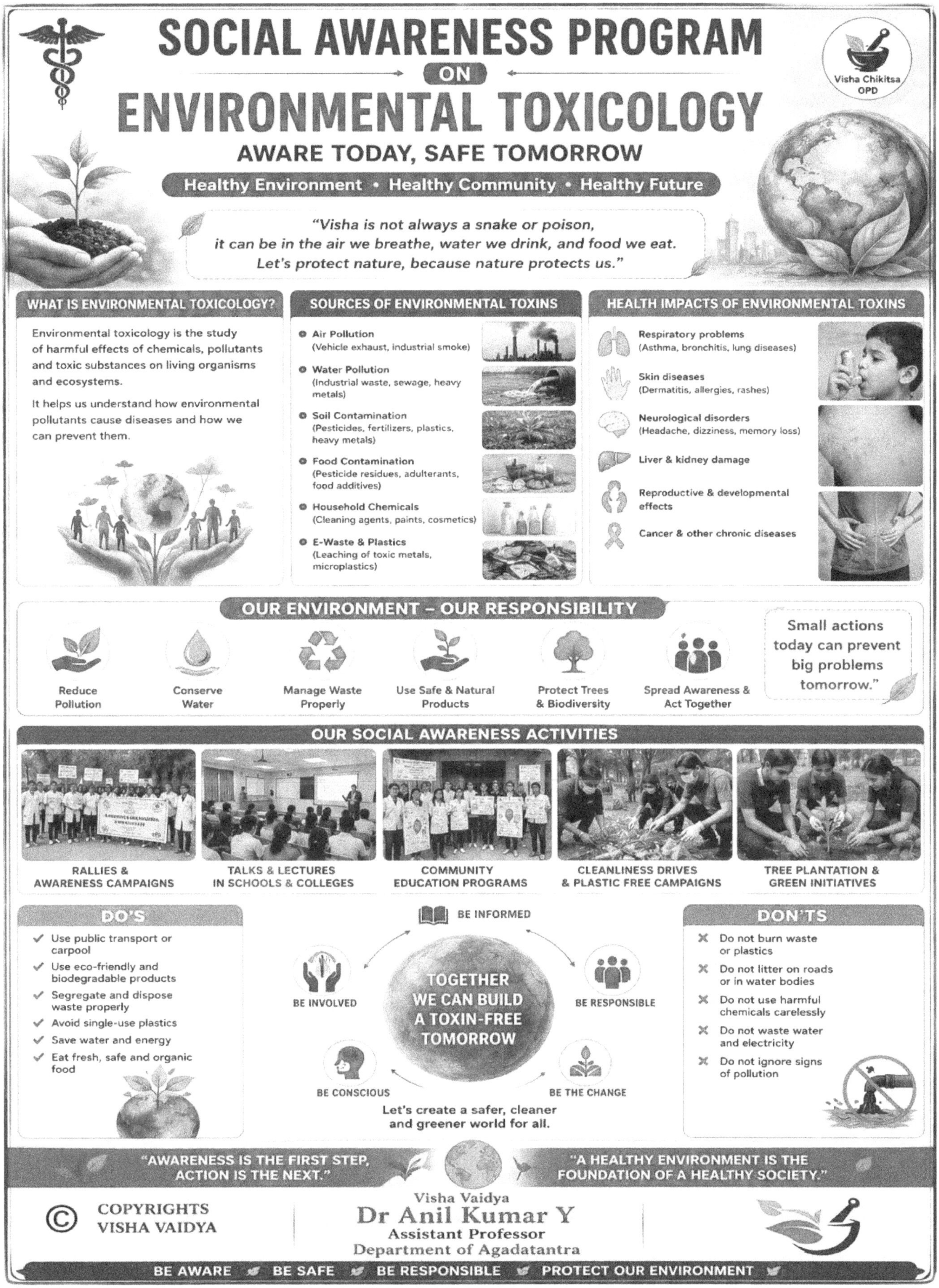
SOCIAL AWARENESS PROGRAM
ON
ENVIRONMENTAL TOXICOLOGY
Visha Chikitsa OPD
AWARE TODAY, SAFE TOMORROW
Healthy Environment • Healthy Community • Healthy Future
"Visha is not always a snake or poison,
it can be in the air we breathe, water we drink, and food we eat.
Let's protect nature, because nature protects us."
WHAT IS ENVIRONMENTAL TOXICOLOGY?
Environmental toxicology is the study of harmful effects of chemicals, pollutants and toxic substances on living organisms and ecosystems.
It helps us understand how environmental pollutants cause diseases and how we can prevent them.
SOURCES OF ENVIRONMENTAL TOXINS
Air Pollution (Vehicle exhaust, industrial smoke)
Water Pollution (Industrial waste, sewage, heavy metals)
Soil Contamination (Pesticides, fertilizers, plastics, heavy metals)
Food Contamination (Pesticide residues, adulterants, food additives)
Household Chemicals (Cleaning agents, paints, cosmetics)
E-Waste & Plastics (Leaching of toxic metals, microplastics)
HEALTH IMPACTS OF ENVIRONMENTAL TOXINS
Respiratory problems (Asthma, bronchitis, lung diseases)
Skin diseases (Dermatitis, allergies, rashes)
Neurological disorders (Headache, dizziness, memory loss)
Liver & kidney damage
Reproductive & developmental effects
Cancer & other chronic diseases
OUR ENVIRONMENT – OUR RESPONSIBILITY
Reduce Pollution
Conserve Water
Manage Waste Properly
Use Safe & Natural Products
Protect Trees & Biodiversity
Spread Awareness & Act Together
Small actions today can prevent big problems tomorrow."
OUR SOCIAL AWARENESS ACTIVITIES
RALLIES & AWARENESS CAMPAIGNS
TALKS & LECTURES IN SCHOOLS & COLLEGES
COMMUNITY EDUCATION PROGRAMS
CLEANLINESS DRIVES & PLASTIC FREE CAMPAIGNS
TREE PLANTATION & GREEN INITIATIVES
DO'S
✓ Use public transport or carpool
✓ Use eco-friendly and biodegradable products
✓ Segregate and dispose waste properly
✓ Avoid single-use plastics
✓ Save water and energy
✓ Eat fresh, safe and organic food
BE INFORMED
BE INVOLVED
BE RESPONSIBLE
BE CONSCIOUS
BE THE CHANGE
TOGETHER WE CAN BUILD A TOXIN-FREE TOMORROW
Let's create a safer, cleaner and greener world for all.
DON'TS
✗ Do not burn waste or plastics
✗ Do not litter on roads or in water bodies
✗ Do not use harmful chemicals carelessly
✗ Do not waste water and electricity
✗ Do not ignore signs of pollution
"AWARENESS IS THE FIRST STEP, ACTION IS THE NEXT."
"A HEALTHY ENVIRONMENT IS THE FOUNDATION OF A HEALTHY SOCIETY."
© COPYRIGHTS VISHA VAIDYA
Visha Vaidya
Dr Anil Kumar Y
Assistant Professor
Department of Agadatantra
BE AWARE BE SAFE BE RESPONSIBLE PROTECT OUR ENVIRONMENT

PRACTICAL NO. 5

ENVIRONMENTAL TOXICOLOGY

Survey Record 1:AIR POLLUTION

Topic:

Date:

Area Surveyed:

Environmental Hazard Identified:

Health Effects:

Preventive Measures:

Student Conclusions:

Faculty Signature

PRACTICAL NO. 5

ENVIRONMENTAL TOXICOLOGY

Survey Record 2: WATER POLLUTION

Topic:

Date:

Area Surveyed:

Environmental Hazard Identified:

Health Effects:

Preventive Measures:

Student Conclusions:

Faculty Signature

PRACTICAL NO. 5

ENVIRONMENTAL TOXICOLOGY

Survey Record 3: SOIL POLLUTION

Topic:

Date:

Area Surveyed:

Environmental Hazard Identified:

Health Effects:

Preventive Measures:

Student Conclusions:

Faculty Signature

PRACTICAL NO. 5

ENVIRONMENTAL TOXICOLOGY

Survey Record 4: SOUND POLLUTION

Topic:

Date:

Area Surveyed:

Environmental Hazard Identified:

Health Effects:

Preventive Measures:

Student Conclusions:

Faculty Signature

PRACTICAL NO. 6

JANGAMA VISHA RECORD

Identification Sheet **Date:**

Animal	Scientific Name	Poison Type	Symptoms	First Aid
Snake				
Scorpion				
Spider				

Animal	Scientific Name	Poison Type	Symptoms	First Aid
Bee				

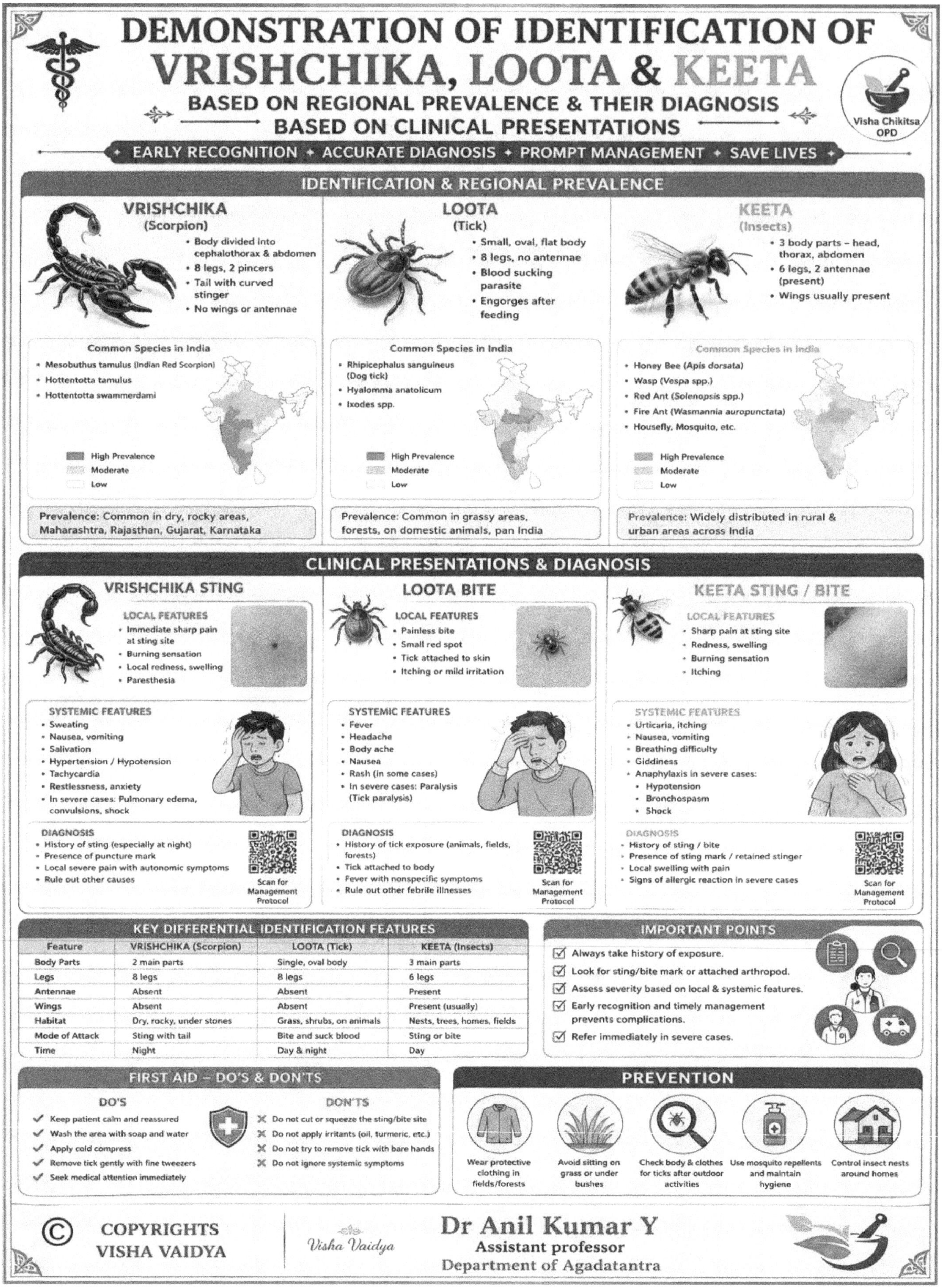

DEMONSTRATION OF IDENTIFICATION OF VRISHCHIKA, LOOTA & KEETA

BASED ON REGIONAL PREVALENCE & THEIR DIAGNOSIS BASED ON CLINICAL PRESENTATIONS

Visha Chikitsa OPD

EARLY RECOGNITION ✦ ACCURATE DIAGNOSIS ✦ PROMPT MANAGEMENT ✦ SAVE LIVES

IDENTIFICATION & REGIONAL PREVALENCE

VRISHCHIKA (Scorpion)

- Body divided into cephalothorax & abdomen
- 8 legs, 2 pincers
- Tail with curved stinger
- No wings or antennae

Common Species in India

- Mesobuthus tamulus (Indian Red Scorpion)
- Hottentotta tamulus
- Hottentotta swammerdami

High Prevalence / Moderate / Low

Prevalence: Common in dry, rocky areas, Maharashtra, Rajasthan, Gujarat, Karnataka

LOOTA (Tick)

- Small, oval, flat body
- 8 legs, no antennae
- Blood sucking parasite
- Engorges after feeding

Common Species in India

- Rhipicephalus sanguineus (Dog tick)
- Hyalomma anatolicum
- Ixodes spp.

High Prevalence / Moderate / Low

Prevalence: Common in grassy areas, forests, on domestic animals, pan India

KEETA (Insects)

- 3 body parts – head, thorax, abdomen
- 6 legs, 2 antennae (present)
- Wings usually present

Common Species in India

- Honey Bee (*Apis dorsata*)
- Wasp (*Vespa* spp.)
- Red Ant (*Solenopsis* spp.)
- Fire Ant (*Wasmannia auropunctata*)
- Housefly, Mosquito, etc.

High Prevalence / Moderate / Low

Prevalence: Widely distributed in rural & urban areas across India

CLINICAL PRESENTATIONS & DIAGNOSIS

VRISHCHIKA STING

LOCAL FEATURES

- Immediate sharp pain at sting site
- Burning sensation
- Local redness, swelling
- Paresthesia

SYSTEMIC FEATURES

- Sweating
- Nausea, vomiting
- Salivation
- Hypertension / Hypotension
- Tachycardia
- Restlessness, anxiety
- In severe cases: Pulmonary edema, convulsions, shock

DIAGNOSIS

- History of sting (especially at night)
- Presence of puncture mark
- Local severe pain with autonomic symptoms
- Rule out other causes

Scan for Management Protocol

LOOTA BITE

LOCAL FEATURES

- Painless bite
- Small red spot
- Tick attached to skin
- Itching or mild irritation

SYSTEMIC FEATURES

- Fever
- Headache
- Body ache
- Nausea
- Rash (in some cases)
- In severe cases: Paralysis (Tick paralysis)

DIAGNOSIS

- History of tick exposure (animals, fields, forests)
- Tick attached to body
- Fever with nonspecific symptoms
- Rule out other febrile illnesses

Scan for Management Protocol

KEETA STING / BITE

LOCAL FEATURES

- Sharp pain at sting site
- Redness, swelling
- Burning sensation
- Itching

SYSTEMIC FEATURES

- Urticaria, itching
- Nausea, vomiting
- Breathing difficulty
- Giddiness
- Anaphylaxis in severe cases:
  - Hypotension
  - Bronchospasm
  - Shock

DIAGNOSIS

- History of sting / bite
- Presence of sting mark / retained stinger
- Local swelling with pain
- Signs of allergic reaction in severe cases

Scan for Management Protocol

KEY DIFFERENTIAL IDENTIFICATION FEATURES

Feature	VRISHCHIKA (Scorpion)	LOOTA (Tick)	KEETA (Insects)
Body Parts	2 main parts	Single, oval body	3 main parts
Legs	8 legs	8 legs	6 legs
Antennae	Absent	Absent	Present
Wings	Absent	Absent	Present (usually)
Habitat	Dry, rocky, under stones	Grass, shrubs, on animals	Nests, trees, homes, fields
Mode of Attack	Sting with tail	Bite and suck blood	Sting or bite
Time	Night	Day & night	Day

IMPORTANT POINTS

- ☑ Always take history of exposure.
- ☑ Look for sting/bite mark or attached arthropod.
- ☑ Assess severity based on local & systemic features.
- ☑ Early recognition and timely management prevents complications.
- ☑ Refer immediately in severe cases.

FIRST AID – DO'S & DON'TS

DO'S

- ✔ Keep patient calm and reassured
- ✔ Wash the area with soap and water
- ✔ Apply cold compress
- ✔ Remove tick gently with fine tweezers
- ✔ Seek medical attention immediately

DON'TS

- ✘ Do not cut or squeeze the sting/bite site
- ✘ Do not apply irritants (oil, turmeric, etc.)
- ✘ Do not try to remove tick with bare hands
- ✘ Do not ignore systemic symptoms

PREVENTION

- Wear protective clothing in fields/forests
- Avoid sitting on grass or under bushes
- Check body & clothes for ticks after outdoor activities
- Use mosquito repellents and maintain hygiene
- Control insect nests around homes

Visha Vaidya

Dr Anil Kumar Y
Assistant professor
Department of Agadatantra

DEMONSTRATION OF THE DIAGNOSIS OF POISONOUS SNAKE BITE CASES

BASED ON LOCAL AND SYSTEMIC CLINICAL PRESENTATIONS

Visha Chikitsa OPD

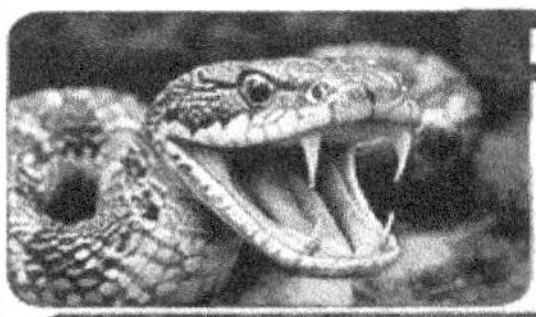

EARLY IDENTIFICATION • PROMPT MANAGEMENT • SAVE LIVES

⚠ **NOTE:** Clinical features may vary depending on the species, amount of venom injected, site of bite, time elapsed and patient's condition.

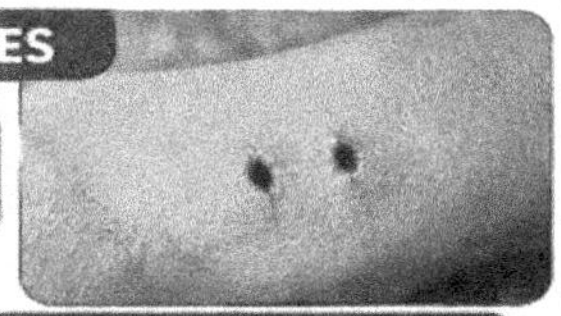

LOCAL CLINICAL PRESENTATIONS (At the Site of Bite)

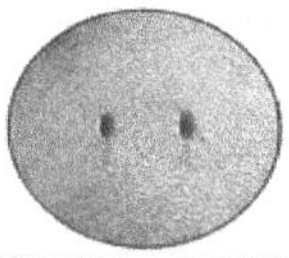

1. FANG MARKS
- One or two puncture wounds (Fang marks)
- May have bleeding or oozing
- Distance between marks varies with species

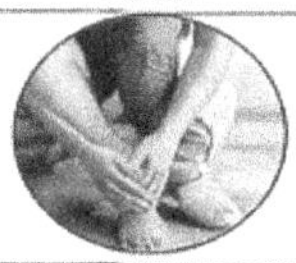

2. PAIN
- Immediate, severe, throbbing pain at the bite site
- Spreads proximally
- Local tenderness

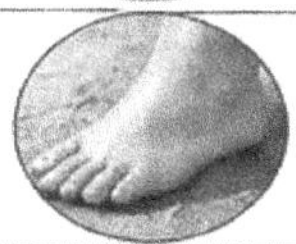

3. SWELLING (EDEMA)
- Local swelling at bite site
- Rapidly progressive
- May extend to whole limb in viper bites

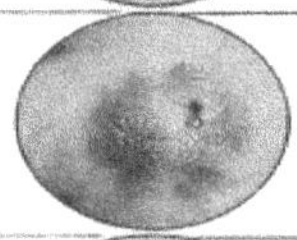

4. LOCAL DISCOLORATION
- Redness, bruising, ecchymosis
- Blister formation
- Necrosis in severe cases

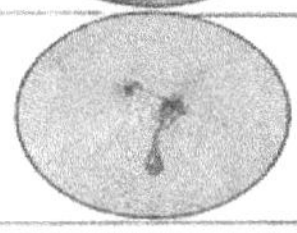

5. LOCAL BLEEDING
- Oozing from bite site
- May be spontaneous or on pressure

SYSTEMIC CLINICAL PRESENTATIONS (In Envenomation)

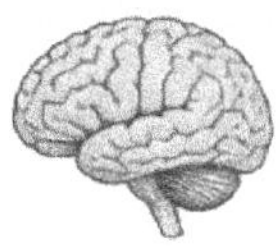

NEUROTOXIC (Eg. Cobra, Krait)
- Ptosis, difficulty in opening eyes
- Diplopia, blurred vision
- Dysarthria, dysphagia
- Respiratory muscle weakness
- Progressive paralysis

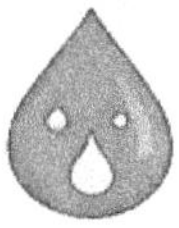

HEMOTOXIC / VASCULOTOXIC (Eg. Russell's viper, Saw-scaled viper)
- Bleeding from gums, nose, bite site
- Hematuria, melena
- Coagulopathy, incoagulable blood
- Shock

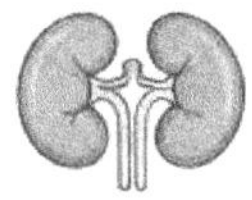

RENAL TOXICITY (Often in Viper bites)
- Oliguria / Anuria
- Hematuria
- Raised serum creatinine, urea
- Acute kidney injury

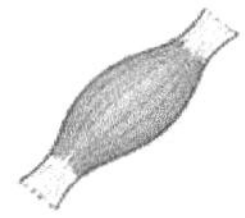

MYOTOXICITY (Rare)
- Muscle pain
- Tenderness
- Raised CK levels
- Myoglobinuria

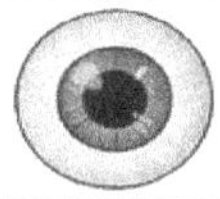

AUTONOMIC MANIFESTATIONS
- Sweating, salivation
- Nausea, vomiting
- Hypotension
- Tachycardia / Bradycardia

DIFFERENTIATING CLINICAL FEATURES OF COMMON POISONOUS SNAKE BITES

Snake Type	Local Signs	Systemic Signs	Other Clues
Cobra (Neurotoxic) 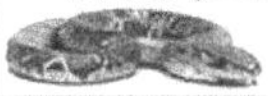	• Mild pain • Minimal swelling	• Ptosis, diplopia • Dysarthria, dysphagia • Respiratory paralysis	• May occur indoors • Slit-like nostrils on hood 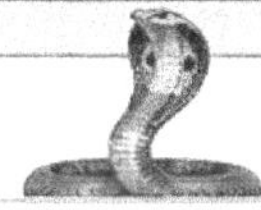
Krait (Neurotoxic) 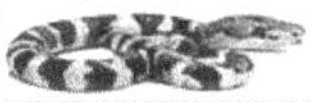	• Painless bite • Minimal swelling	• Similar to cobra • Late onset paralysis • No local reaction	• Nocturnal bite • Bite may be unnoticed 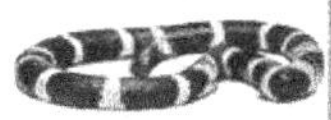
Russell's Viper (Hemotoxic) 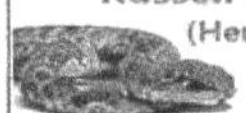	• Severe pain • Rapid swelling • Blister, necrosis	• Bleeding manifestations • Coagulopathy • Shock, AKI	• Oval / round pupils • Found in fields 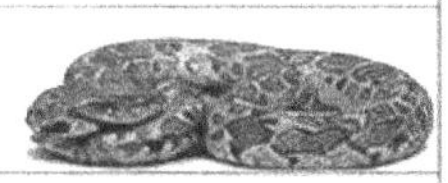
Saw-scaled Viper (Hemotoxic) 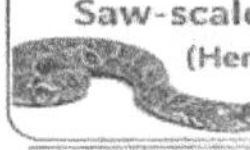	• Severe pain • Swelling • Ecchymosis	• Bleeding • Hemolysis • Shock	• Small size • Harsh, sawing sound when moving 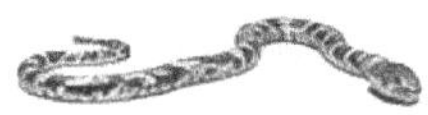

DIAGNOSTIC APPROACH

- ☑ Detailed history (time, place, activity, snake seen or not)
- ☑ Examination of local signs (fang marks, swelling, pain)
- ☑ Assessment of systemic signs (neuro, bleeding, renal, etc.)
- ☑ Lab investigations:
  - 20WBCT, BT, CT, INR
  - Serum creatinine, urea, electrolytes
  - Urine routine & microscopy
  - CK level (if indicated)
- ☑ Continuous monitoring of vital signs

EMERGENCY MANAGEMENT SUMMARY

- Early recognition of envenomation
- Immediate first aid & immobilization
- Prompt administration of ASV
- Supportive management
- Continuous monitoring & referral

FIRST AID - DO'S & DON'TS

DO'S
- ✔ Keep the patient calm and reassured
- ✔ Immobilize the limb (below heart level)
- ✔ Remove tight ornaments
- ✔ Rush to nearest hospital immediately

DON'TS
- ✖ Do not cut, suck, or squeeze the bite
- ✖ Do not apply tourniquet
- ✖ Do not give alcohol, stimulants or food
- ✖ Do not waste time on traditional methods

Dr Anil Kumar Y
Assistant professor
Department of Agadatantra

IDENTIFY EARLY • TREAT PROMPTLY • PREVENT COMPLICATIONS • SAVE LIVES

Difference between Poisonous and Non-Poisoous Snake

Observation Table

Sl. No.	Feature	Poisonous Snake	Non-Poisonous Snake
1	Venom Glands	Present	Absent
2	Fangs	Present, specialized for venom injection	Absent or not specialized
3	Bite Mark	Usually two distinct fang marks	Multiple small teeth marks
4	Venom	Present	Absent
5	Effect of Bite	Causes envenomation and systemic symptoms	Usually harmless except local injury
6	Head Shape	Often broader than neck (not always)	Usually not distinct from neck
7	Tail	May be short and abruptly tapering	Usually long and gradually tapering
8	Danger to Humans	Potentially fatal	Generally harmless
9	Medical Importance	Requires emergency treatment and ASV in indicated cases	Usually requires wound care only
10	Examples	Cobra, Krait, Russell's Viper, Saw-scaled Viper	Rat Snake, Python, Trinket Snake, Sand Boa

---

Common Poisonous Snakes of India (Big Four)

1. Indian Cobra (*Naja naja*)
2. Common Krait (*Bungarus caeruleus*)
3. Russell's Viper (*Daboia russelii*)
4. Saw-scaled Viper (*Echis carinatus*)

Common Non-Poisonous Snakes

1. Rat Snake (*Ptyas mucosa*)
2. Indian Rock Python (*Python molurus*)
3. Sand Boa (*Eryx johnii*)
4. Trinket Snake (*Coelognathus helena*)

IDENTIFICATION OF POISONOUS AND NON POISONOUS SNAKES

Learn to Identify... Stay Safe... Save Lives...

POISONOUS SNAKES (Venomous)

These snakes have venom glands and fangs to inject venom. Handle with extreme caution. Seek medical help immediately in case of a bite.

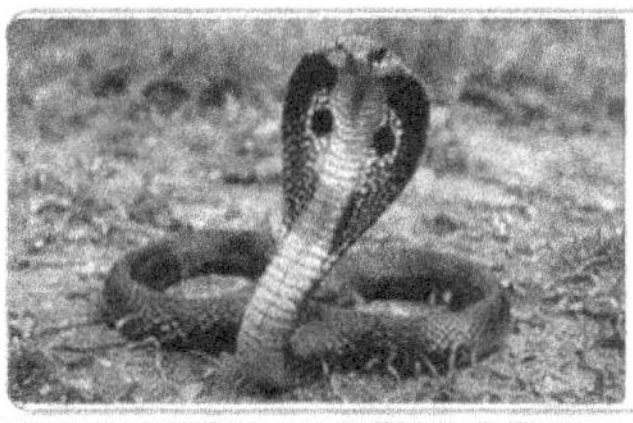

1. INDIAN COBRA

(Naja naja)

- Hood spread when threatened
- "Spectacle" mark on hood
- Found in fields, houses, wooded areas
- Venom: Neurotoxic

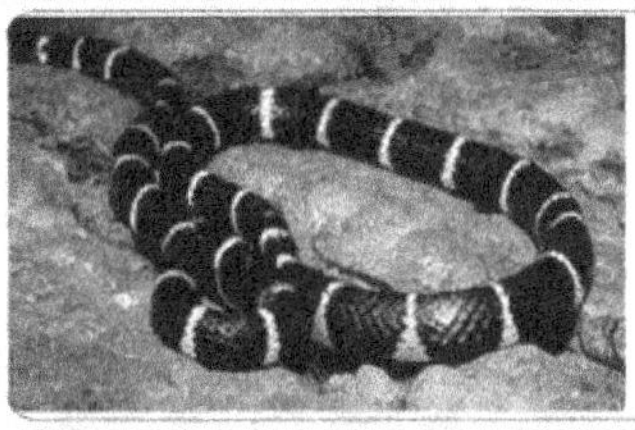

2. COMMON KRAIT

(Bungarus caeruleus)

- Shiny black or blue-black body with white bands
- Nocturnal, found in houses, fields
- Venom: Neurotoxic

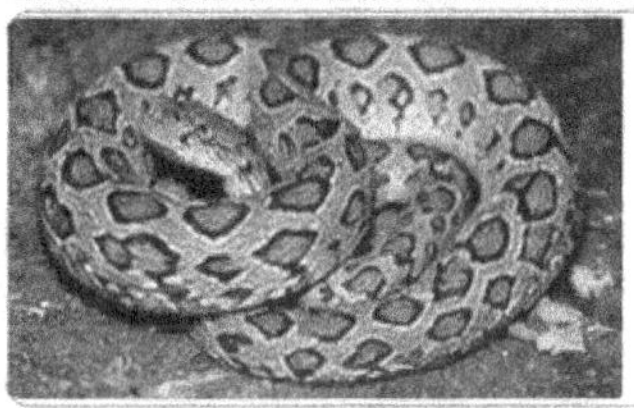

3. RUSSELL'S VIPER

(Daboia russelii)

- Heavy body with three rows of oval spots
- Found in fields, grasslands
- Venom: Hemotoxic

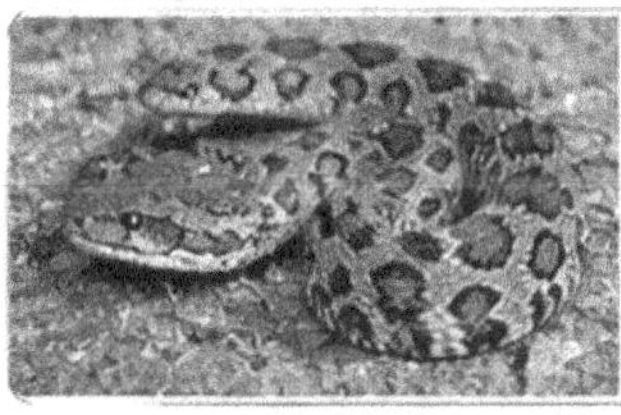

4. SAW-SCALED VIPER

(Echis carinatus)

- Small size, rough scales
- Produces a saw-like sound by rubbing scales
- Found in dry, sandy areas
- Venom: Hemotoxic

KEY IDENTIFICATION FEATURES OF POISONOUS SNAKES

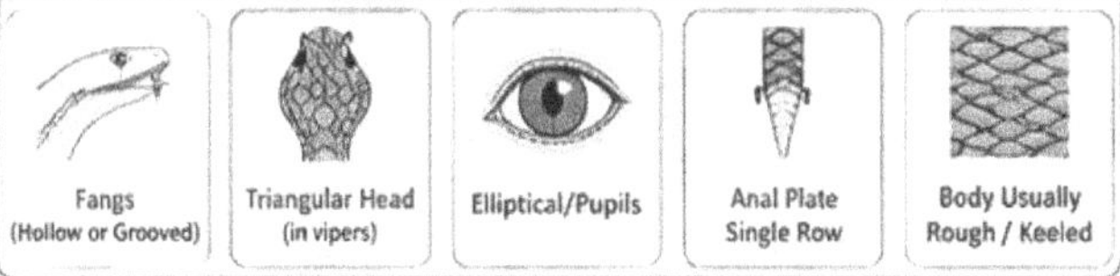
Fangs
(Hollow or Grooved)
Triangular Head
(in vipers)
Elliptical/Pupils
Anal Plate
Single Row
Body Usually
Rough / Keeled

DO NOT TRY TO KILL OR CATCH THE SNAKE

Stay calm, move away slowly and seek medical help immediately.

NON POISONOUS SNAKES (Non Venomous)

These snakes do not have venom glands or fangs. Generally harmless and help in controlling pests.

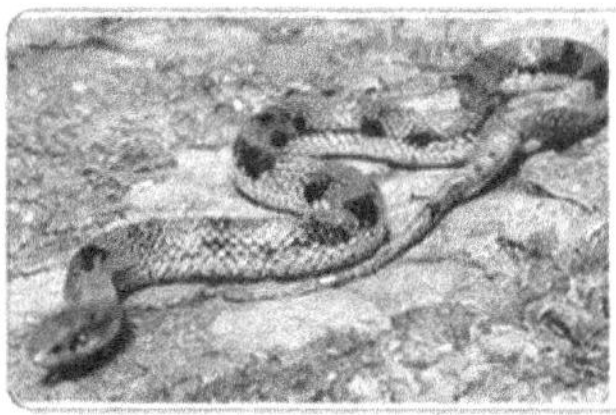

1. INDIAN RAT SNAKE

(Ptyas mucosa)

- Long, slender body
- Brown or grey with black markings
- Excellent climber
- Harmless

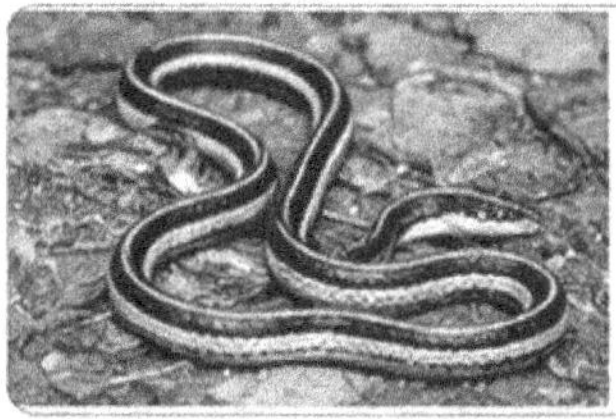

2. TRINKET SNAKE

(Coelognathus helena)

- Brown or olive with yellow/white stripes
- Small, active, avoids humans
- Harmless

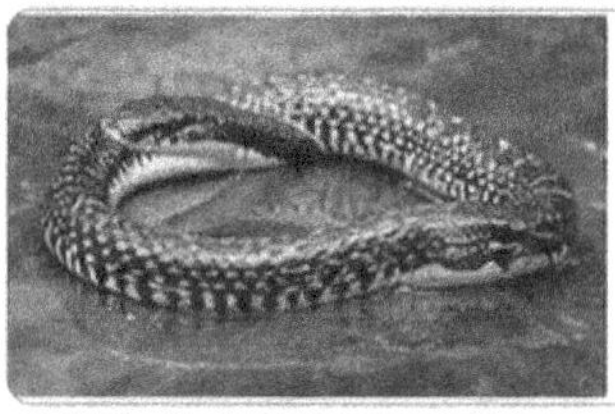

3. CHECKERED KEELBACK

(Fowlea piscator)

- Olive or brown with checkered pattern
- Found near water bodies
- Harmless

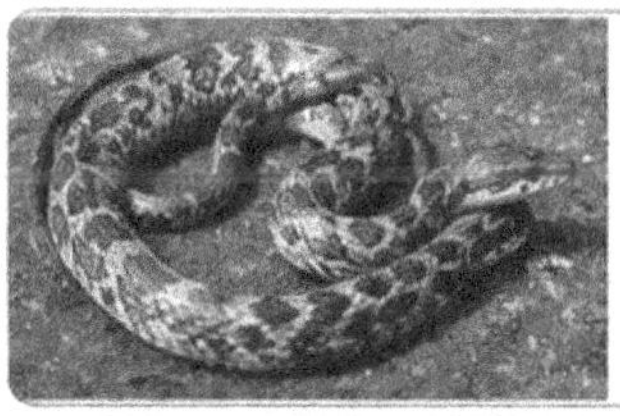

4. COMMON WOLF SNAKE

(Lycodon aulicus)

- Brown with white or yellow cross bands
- Non-aggressive
- Harmless

KEY IDENTIFICATION FEATURES OF NON POISONOUS SNAKES

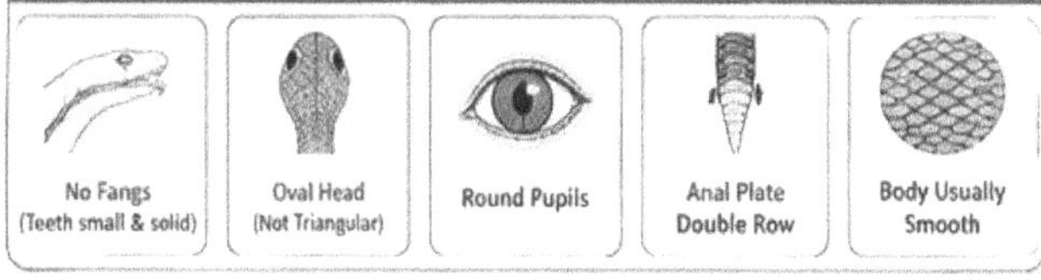

GENERAL POINTS TO REMEMBER

- Do not rely on color alone for identification.
- When in doubt, consider the snake to be poisonous.
- Most snakes are harmless and play an important role in nature.
- Always respect snakes and their habitat.

Dr Anil Kumar Y
Assistant professor
Department of Agadatantra

PRACTICAL NO. 6

DERMATOLOGICAL MANIFESTATIONS OF VISHA

BITES/STINGS

Case No:01

Date:

Patient Details

Name::

Age::

Sex:

Address:

Occupation:

Chief Complaints:

History of Present Illness:

Exposure History:

Nidana:

Examination:

Samprapti:

Differential Diagnosis:

Diagnosis:

Treatment Given

Outcome

Discussion

Faculty Signature

PRACTICAL NO. 6

DERMATOLOGICAL MANIFESTATIONS OF VISHA

BITES/STINGS

Case No:02

Date:

Patient Details

Name::

Age::

Sex:

Address:

Occupation:

Chief Complaints:

History of Present Illness:

Exposure History:

Nidana:

Examination:

Samprapti:

Differential Diagnosis:

Diagnosis:

Treatment Given

Outcome

Discussion

Faculty Signature

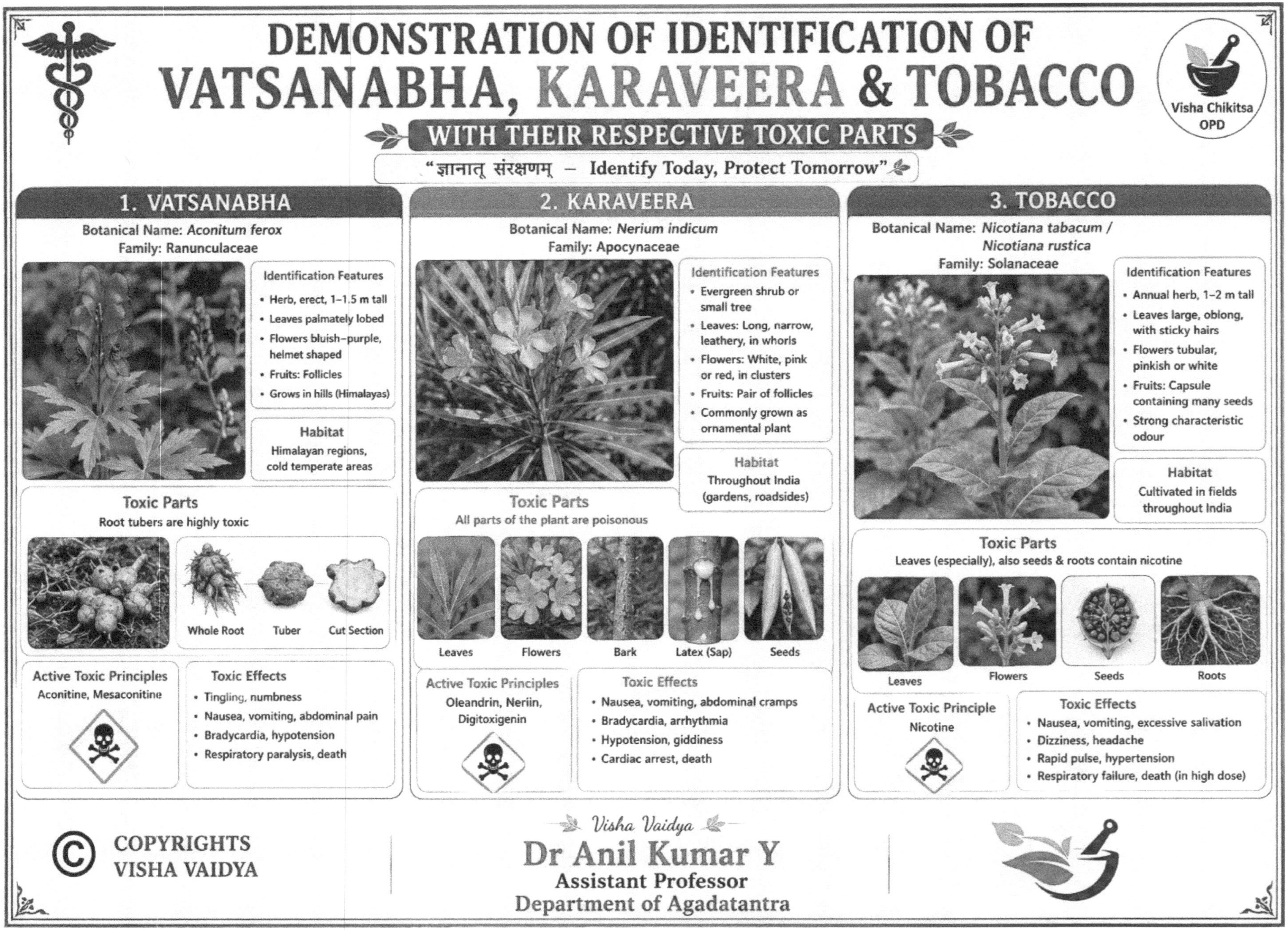
DEMONSTRATION OF IDENTIFICATION OF
VATSANABHA, KARAVEERA & TOBACCO
WITH THEIR RESPECTIVE TOXIC PARTS
"ज्ञानात् संरक्षणम् – Identify Today, Protect Tomorrow"
Visha Chikitsa OPD
1. VATSANABHA
Botanical Name: Aconitum ferox
Family: Ranunculaceae
Identification Features
• Herb, erect, 1–1.5 m tall
• Leaves palmately lobed
• Flowers bluish-purple, helmet shaped
• Fruits: Follicles
• Grows in hills (Himalayas)
Habitat
Himalayan regions, cold temperate areas
Toxic Parts
Root tubers are highly toxic
Whole Root
Tuber
Cut Section
Active Toxic Principles
Aconitine, Mesaconitine
Toxic Effects
• Tingling, numbness
• Nausea, vomiting, abdominal pain
• Bradycardia, hypotension
• Respiratory paralysis, death
2. KARAVEERA
Botanical Name: Nerium indicum
Family: Apocynaceae
Identification Features
• Evergreen shrub or small tree
• Leaves: Long, narrow, leathery, in whorls
• Flowers: White, pink or red, in clusters
• Fruits: Pair of follicles
• Commonly grown as ornamental plant
Habitat
Throughout India (gardens, roadsides)
Toxic Parts
All parts of the plant are poisonous
Leaves
Flowers
Bark
Latex (Sap)
Seeds
Active Toxic Principles
Oleandrin, Neriin, Digitoxigenin
Toxic Effects
• Nausea, vomiting, abdominal cramps
• Bradycardia, arrhythmia
• Hypotension, giddiness
• Cardiac arrest, death
3. TOBACCO
Botanical Name: Nicotiana tabacum / Nicotiana rustica
Family: Solanaceae
Identification Features
• Annual herb, 1–2 m tall
• Leaves large, oblong, with sticky hairs
• Flowers tubular, pinkish or white
• Fruits: Capsule containing many seeds
• Strong characteristic odour
Habitat
Cultivated in fields throughout India
Toxic Parts
Leaves (especially), also seeds & roots contain nicotine
Leaves
Flowers
Seeds
Roots
Active Toxic Principle
Nicotine
Toxic Effects
• Nausea, vomiting, excessive salivation
• Dizziness, headache
• Rapid pulse, hypertension
• Respiratory failure, death (in high dose)
© COPYRIGHTS VISHA VAIDYA
Visha Vaidya
Dr Anil Kumar Y
Assistant Professor
Department of Agadatantra

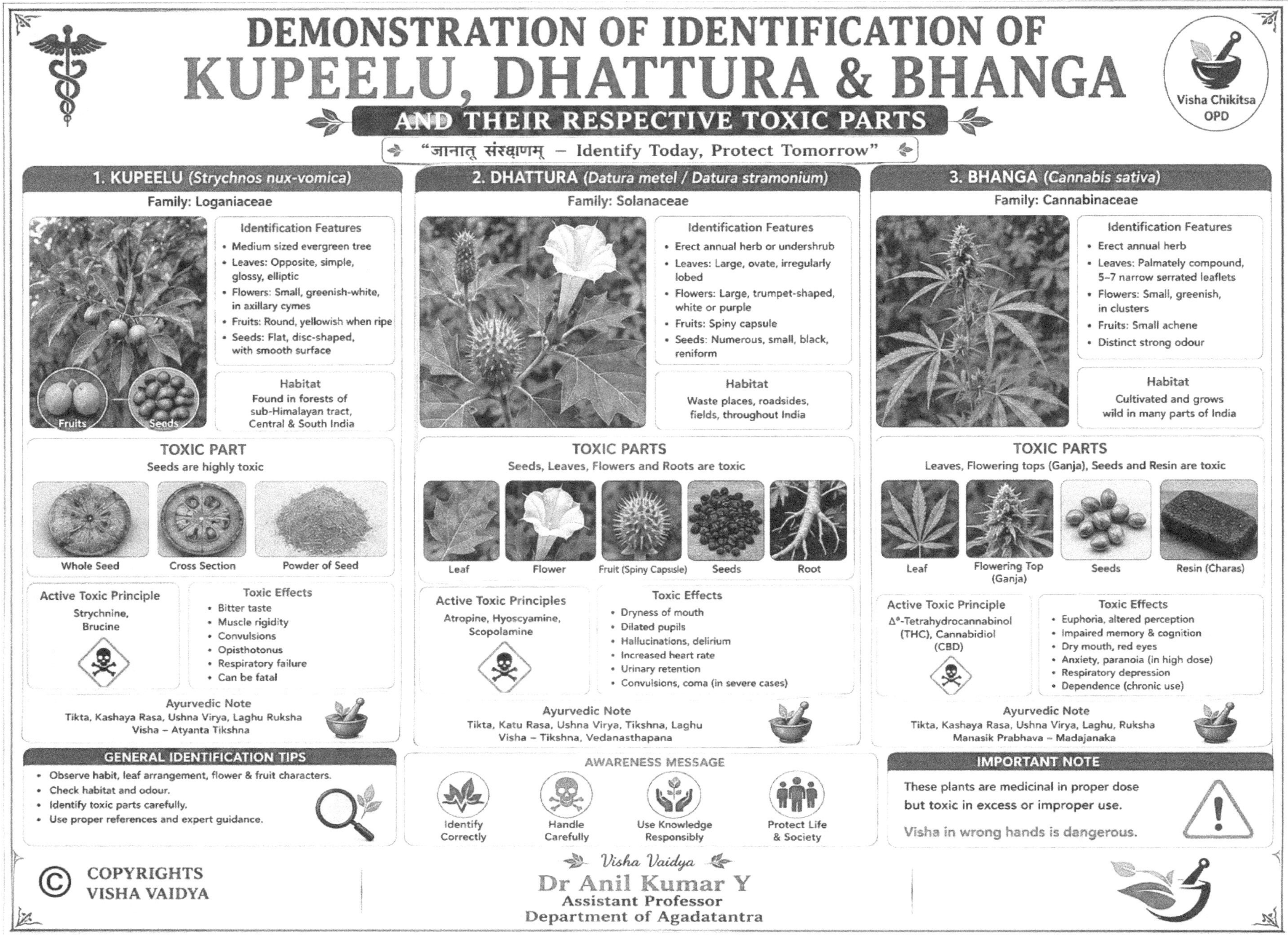
DEMONSTRATION OF IDENTIFICATION OF
KUPEELU, DHATTURA & BHANGA
AND THEIR RESPECTIVE TOXIC PARTS
"जानातु संरक्षणम् – Identify Today, Protect Tomorrow"
Visha Chikitsa OPD
1. KUPEELU (Strychnos nux-vomica)
Family: Loganiaceae
Fruits
Seeds
Identification Features
• Medium sized evergreen tree
• Leaves: Opposite, simple, glossy, elliptic
• Flowers: Small, greenish-white, in axillary cymes
• Fruits: Round, yellowish when ripe
• Seeds: Flat, disc-shaped, with smooth surface
Habitat
Found in forests of sub-Himalayan tract, Central & South India
TOXIC PART
Seeds are highly toxic
Whole Seed
Cross Section
Powder of Seed
Active Toxic Principle
Strychnine, Brucine
Toxic Effects
• Bitter taste
• Muscle rigidity
• Convulsions
• Opisthotonus
• Respiratory failure
• Can be fatal
Ayurvedic Note
Tikta, Kashaya Rasa, Ushna Virya, Laghu Ruksha
Visha – Atyanta Tikshna
2. DHATTURA (Datura metel / Datura stramonium)
Family: Solanaceae
Identification Features
• Erect annual herb or undershrub
• Leaves: Large, ovate, irregularly lobed
• Flowers: Large, trumpet-shaped, white or purple
• Fruits: Spiny capsule
• Seeds: Numerous, small, black, reniform
Habitat
Waste places, roadsides, fields, throughout India
TOXIC PARTS
Seeds, Leaves, Flowers and Roots are toxic
Leaf
Flower
Fruit (Spiny Capsule)
Seeds
Root
Active Toxic Principles
Atropine, Hyoscyamine, Scopolamine
Toxic Effects
• Dryness of mouth
• Dilated pupils
• Hallucinations, delirium
• Increased heart rate
• Urinary retention
• Convulsions, coma (in severe cases)
Ayurvedic Note
Tikta, Katu Rasa, Ushna Virya, Tikshna, Laghu
Visha – Tikshna, Vedanasthapana
3. BHANGA (Cannabis sativa)
Family: Cannabinaceae
Identification Features
• Erect annual herb
• Leaves: Palmately compound, 5–7 narrow serrated leaflets
• Flowers: Small, greenish, in clusters
• Fruits: Small achene
• Distinct strong odour
Habitat
Cultivated and grows wild in many parts of India
TOXIC PARTS
Leaves, Flowering tops (Ganja), Seeds and Resin are toxic
Leaf
Flowering Top (Ganja)
Seeds
Resin (Charas)
Active Toxic Principle
Δ⁹-Tetrahydrocannabinol (THC), Cannabidiol (CBD)
Toxic Effects
• Euphoria, altered perception
• Impaired memory & cognition
• Dry mouth, red eyes
• Anxiety, paranoia (in high dose)
• Respiratory depression
• Dependence (chronic use)
Ayurvedic Note
Tikta, Kashaya Rasa, Ushna Virya, Laghu, Ruksha
Manasik Prabhava – Madajanaka
GENERAL IDENTIFICATION TIPS
• Observe habit, leaf arrangement, flower & fruit characters.
• Check habitat and odour.
• Identify toxic parts carefully.
• Use proper references and expert guidance.
AWARENESS MESSAGE
Identify Correctly
Handle Carefully
Use Knowledge Responsibly
Protect Life & Society
IMPORTANT NOTE
These plants are medicinal in proper dose but toxic in excess or improper use.
Visha in wrong hands is dangerous.
© COPYRIGHTS VISHA VAIDYA
Visha Vaidya
Dr Anil Kumar Y
Assistant Professor
Department of Agadatantra

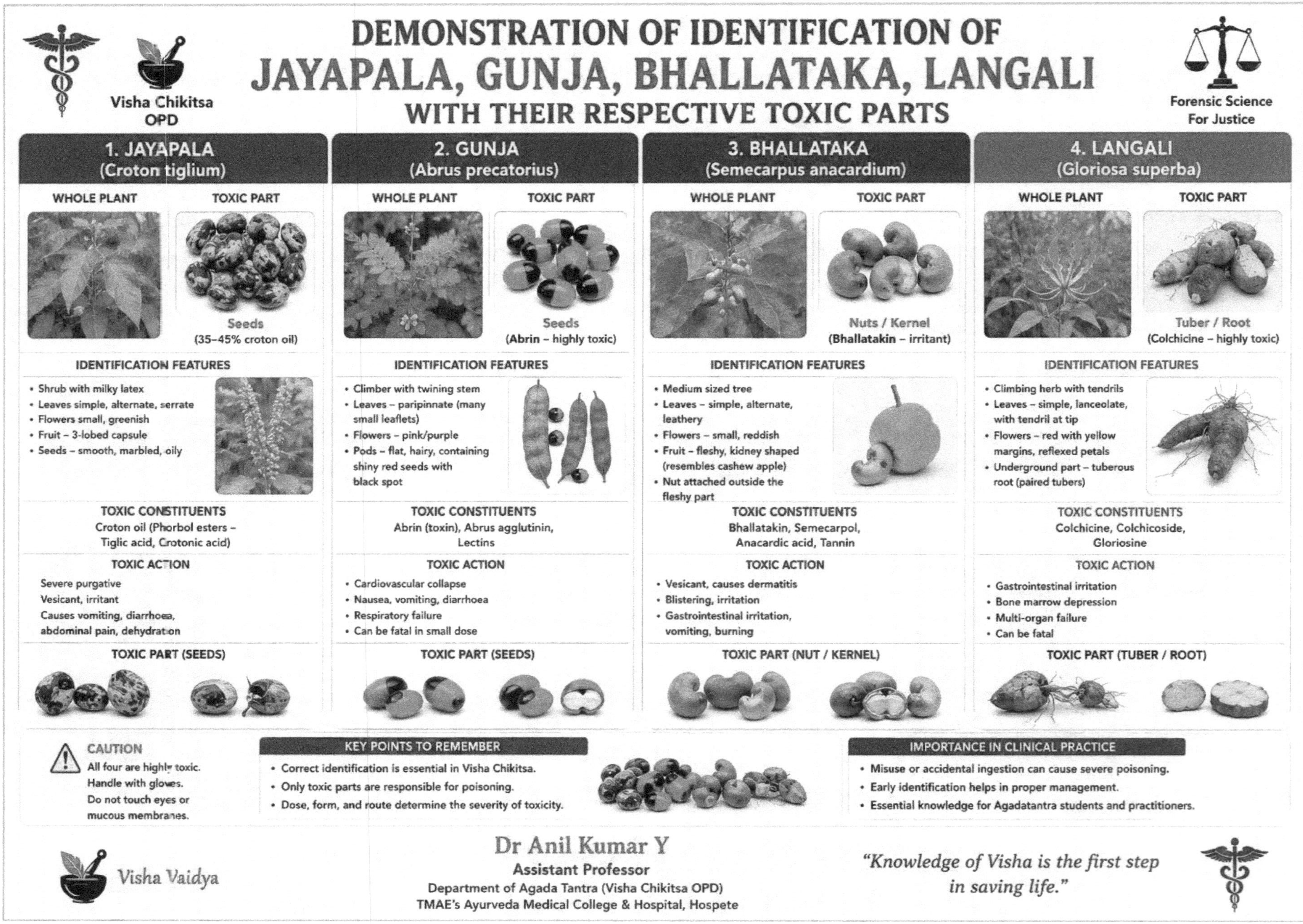

Visha Chikitsa OPD
DEMONSTRATION OF IDENTIFICATION OF
JAYAPALA, GUNJA, BHALLATAKA, LANGALI
WITH THEIR RESPECTIVE TOXIC PARTS
Forensic Science For Justice
1. JAYAPALA (Croton tiglium)
WHOLE PLANT
TOXIC PART
Seeds (35–45% croton oil)
IDENTIFICATION FEATURES
• Shrub with milky latex
• Leaves simple, alternate, serrate
• Flowers small, greenish
• Fruit – 3-lobed capsule
• Seeds – smooth, marbled, oily
TOXIC CONSTITUENTS
Croton oil (Phorbol esters – Tiglic acid, Crotonic acid)
TOXIC ACTION
Severe purgative
Vesicant, irritant
Causes vomiting, diarrhoea, abdominal pain, dehydration
TOXIC PART (SEEDS)
2. GUNJA (Abrus precatorius)
WHOLE PLANT
TOXIC PART
Seeds (Abrin – highly toxic)
IDENTIFICATION FEATURES
• Climber with twining stem
• Leaves – paripinnate (many small leaflets)
• Flowers – pink/purple
• Pods – flat, hairy, containing shiny red seeds with black spot
TOXIC CONSTITUENTS
Abrin (toxin), Abrus agglutinin, Lectins
TOXIC ACTION
• Cardiovascular collapse
• Nausea, vomiting, diarrhoea
• Respiratory failure
• Can be fatal in small dose
TOXIC PART (SEEDS)
3. BHALLATAKA (Semecarpus anacardium)
WHOLE PLANT
TOXIC PART
Nuts / Kernel (Bhallatakin – irritant)
IDENTIFICATION FEATURES
• Medium sized tree
• Leaves – simple, alternate, leathery
• Flowers – small, reddish
• Fruit – fleshy, kidney shaped (resembles cashew apple)
• Nut attached outside the fleshy part
TOXIC CONSTITUENTS
Bhallatakin, Semecarpol, Anacardic acid, Tannin
TOXIC ACTION
• Vesicant, causes dermatitis
• Blistering, irritation
• Gastrointestinal irritation, vomiting, burning
TOXIC PART (NUT / KERNEL)
4. LANGALI (Gloriosa superba)
WHOLE PLANT
TOXIC PART
Tuber / Root (Colchicine – highly toxic)
IDENTIFICATION FEATURES
• Climbing herb with tendrils
• Leaves – simple, lanceolate, with tendril at tip
• Flowers – red with yellow margins, reflexed petals
• Underground part – tuberous root (paired tubers)
TOXIC CONSTITUENTS
Colchicine, Colchicoside, Gloriosine
TOXIC ACTION
• Gastrointestinal irritation
• Bone marrow depression
• Multi-organ failure
• Can be fatal
TOXIC PART (TUBER / ROOT)
CAUTION
All four are highly toxic. Handle with gloves. Do not touch eyes or mucous membranes.
KEY POINTS TO REMEMBER
• Correct identification is essential in Visha Chikitsa.
• Only toxic parts are responsible for poisoning.
• Dose, form, and route determine the severity of toxicity.
IMPORTANCE IN CLINICAL PRACTICE
• Misuse or accidental ingestion can cause severe poisoning.
• Early identification helps in proper management.
• Essential knowledge for Agadatantra students and practitioners.
Visha Vaidya
Dr Anil Kumar Y
Assistant Professor
Department of Agada Tantra (Visha Chikitsa OPD)
TMAE's Ayurveda Medical College & Hospital, Hospete
"Knowledge of Visha is the first step in saving life."

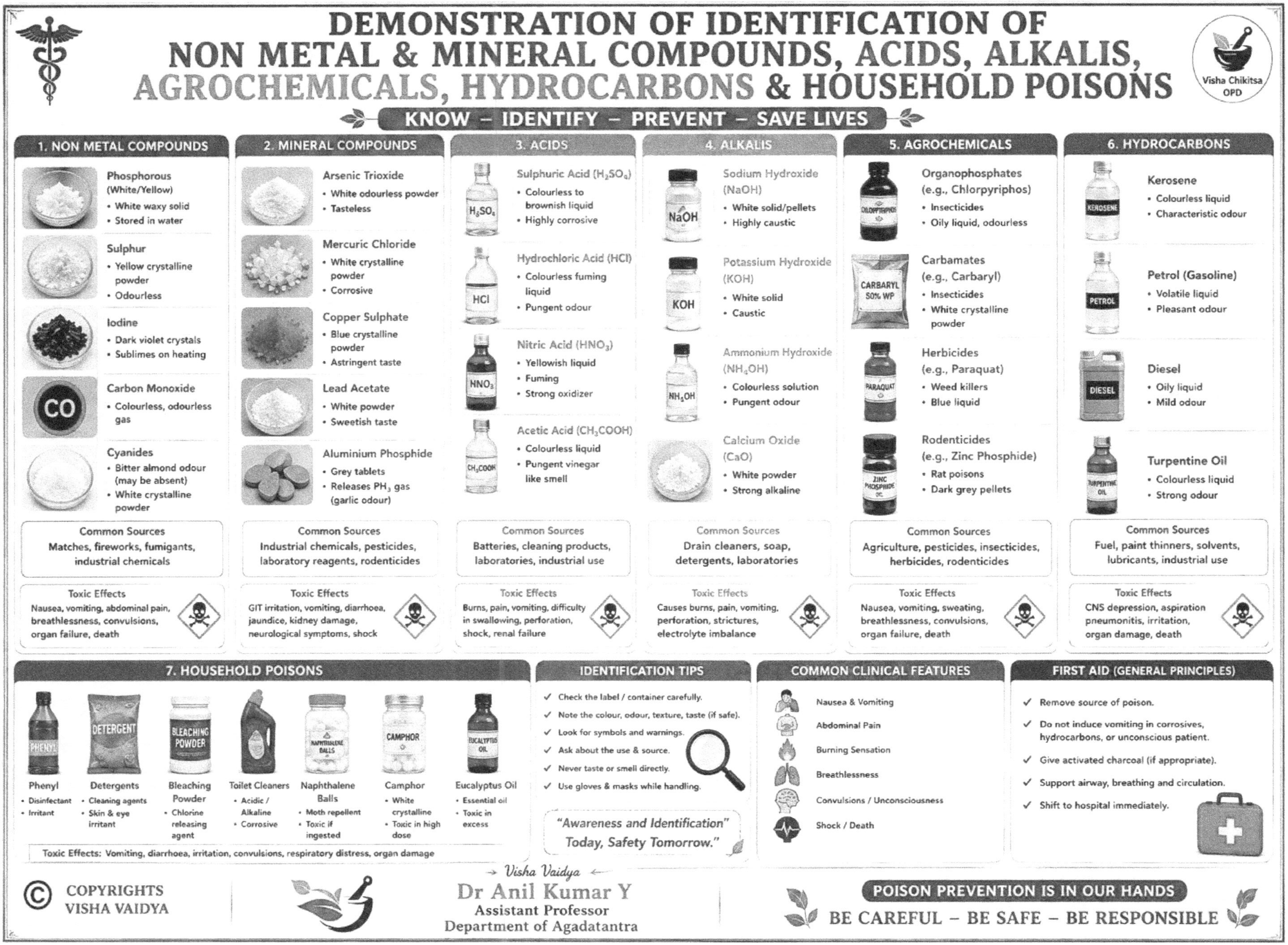
DEMONSTRATION OF IDENTIFICATION OF
NON METAL & MINERAL COMPOUNDS, ACIDS, ALKALIS,
AGROCHEMICALS, HYDROCARBONS & HOUSEHOLD POISONS
Visha Chikitsa OPD
KNOW – IDENTIFY – PREVENT – SAVE LIVES
1. NON METAL COMPOUNDS
Phosphorous (White/Yellow)
• White waxy solid
• Stored in water
Sulphur
• Yellow crystalline powder
• Odourless
Iodine
• Dark violet crystals
• Sublimes on heating
CO
Carbon Monoxide
• Colourless, odourless gas
Cyanides
• Bitter almond odour (may be absent)
• White crystalline powder
Common Sources
Matches, fireworks, fumigants, industrial chemicals
Toxic Effects
Nausea, vomiting, abdominal pain, breathlessness, convulsions, organ failure, death
2. MINERAL COMPOUNDS
Arsenic Trioxide
• White odourless powder
• Tasteless
Mercuric Chloride
• White crystalline powder
• Corrosive
Copper Sulphate
• Blue crystalline powder
• Astringent taste
Lead Acetate
• White powder
• Sweetish taste
Aluminium Phosphide
• Grey tablets
• Releases PH_3 gas (garlic odour)
Common Sources
Industrial chemicals, pesticides, laboratory reagents, rodenticides
Toxic Effects
GIT irritation, vomiting, diarrhoea, jaundice, kidney damage, neurological symptoms, shock
3. ACIDS
H_2SO_4
Sulphuric Acid (H_2SO_4)
• Colourless to brownish liquid
• Highly corrosive
HCl
Hydrochloric Acid (HCl)
• Colourless fuming liquid
• Pungent odour
HNO_3
Nitric Acid (HNO_3)
• Yellowish liquid
• Fuming
• Strong oxidizer
CH_3COOH
Acetic Acid (CH_3COOH)
• Colourless liquid
• Pungent vinegar like smell
Common Sources
Batteries, cleaning products, laboratories, industrial use
Toxic Effects
Burns, pain, vomiting, difficulty in swallowing, perforation, shock, renal failure
4. ALKALIS
NaOH
Sodium Hydroxide (NaOH)
• White solid/pellets
• Highly caustic
KOH
Potassium Hydroxide (KOH)
• White solid
• Caustic
NH_4OH
Ammonium Hydroxide (NH_4OH)
• Colourless solution
• Pungent odour
Calcium Oxide (CaO)
• White powder
• Strong alkaline
Common Sources
Drain cleaners, soap, detergents, laboratories
Toxic Effects
Causes burns, pain, vomiting, perforation, strictures, electrolyte imbalance
5. AGROCHEMICALS
CHLORPYRIPHOS
Organophosphates (e.g., Chlorpyriphos)
• Insecticides
• Oily liquid, odourless
CARBARYL 50% WP
Carbamates (e.g., Carbaryl)
• Insecticides
• White crystalline powder
PARAQUAT
Herbicides (e.g., Paraquat)
• Weed killers
• Blue liquid
ZINC PHOSPHIDE
Rodenticides (e.g., Zinc Phosphide)
• Rat poisons
• Dark grey pellets
Common Sources
Agriculture, pesticides, insecticides, herbicides, rodenticides
Toxic Effects
Nausea, vomiting, sweating, breathlessness, convulsions, organ failure, death
6. HYDROCARBONS
KEROSENE
Kerosene
• Colourless liquid
• Characteristic odour
PETROL
Petrol (Gasoline)
• Volatile liquid
• Pleasant odour
DIESEL
Diesel
• Oily liquid
• Mild odour
TURPENTINE OIL
Turpentine Oil
• Colourless liquid
• Strong odour
Common Sources
Fuel, paint thinners, solvents, lubricants, industrial use
Toxic Effects
CNS depression, aspiration pneumonitis, irritation, organ damage, death
7. HOUSEHOLD POISONS
PHENYL
DETERGENT
BLEACHING POWDER
NAPHTHALENE BALLS
CAMPHOR
EUCALYPTUS OIL
Phenyl
• Disinfectant
• Irritant
Detergents
• Cleaning agents
• Skin & eye irritant
Bleaching Powder
• Chlorine releasing agent
Toilet Cleaners
• Acidic / Alkaline
• Corrosive
Naphthalene Balls
• Moth repellent
• Toxic if ingested
Camphor
• White crystalline
• Toxic in high dose
Eucalyptus Oil
• Essential oil
• Toxic in excess
Toxic Effects: Vomiting, diarrhoea, irritation, convulsions, respiratory distress, organ damage
IDENTIFICATION TIPS
✓ Check the label / container carefully.
✓ Note the colour, odour, texture, taste (if safe).
✓ Look for symbols and warnings.
✓ Ask about the use & source.
✓ Never taste or smell directly.
✓ Use gloves & masks while handling.
"Awareness and Identification" Today, Safety Tomorrow."
COMMON CLINICAL FEATURES
Nausea & Vomiting
Abdominal Pain
Burning Sensation
Breathlessness
Convulsions / Unconsciousness
Shock / Death
FIRST AID (GENERAL PRINCIPLES)
✓ Remove source of poison.
✓ Do not induce vomiting in corrosives, hydrocarbons, or unconscious patient.
✓ Give activated charcoal (if appropriate).
✓ Support airway, breathing and circulation.
✓ Shift to hospital immediately.
© COPYRIGHTS VISHA VAIDYA
→ Visha Vaidya ←
Dr Anil Kumar Y
Assistant Professor
Department of Agadatantra
POISON PREVENTION IS IN OUR HANDS
BE CAREFUL – BE SAFE – BE RESPONSIBLE

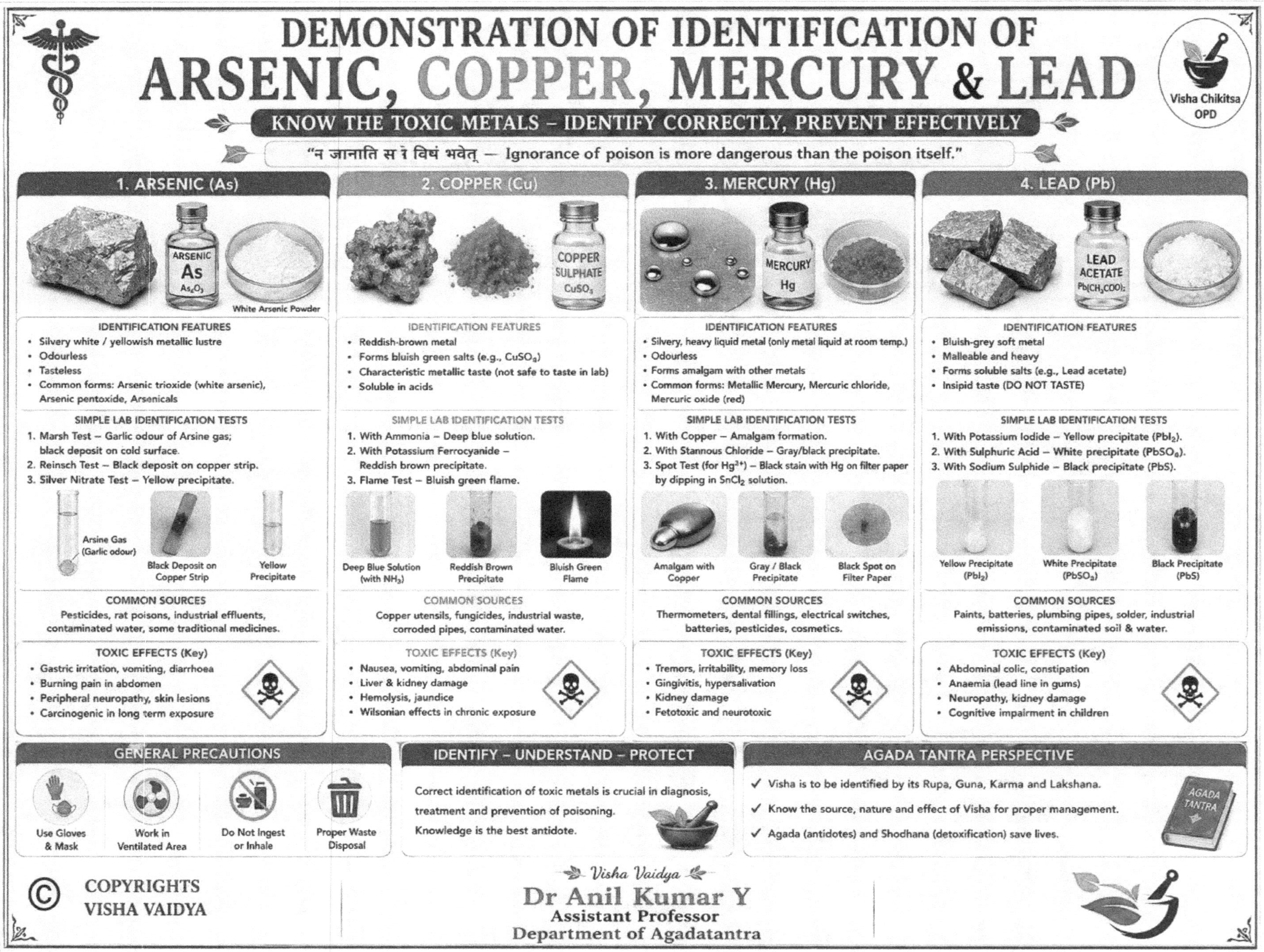
DEMONSTRATION OF IDENTIFICATION OF
ARSENIC, COPPER, MERCURY & LEAD
Visha Chikitsa OPD
KNOW THE TOXIC METALS – IDENTIFY CORRECTLY, PREVENT EFFECTIVELY
"न जानाति स रे विषं भवेत् – Ignorance of poison is more dangerous than the poison itself."
1. ARSENIC (As)
ARSENIC As As_2O_3
White Arsenic Powder
IDENTIFICATION FEATURES
• Silvery white / yellowish metallic lustre
• Odourless
• Tasteless
• Common forms: Arsenic trioxide (white arsenic), Arsenic pentoxide, Arsenicals
SIMPLE LAB IDENTIFICATION TESTS
1. Marsh Test – Garlic odour of Arsine gas; black deposit on cold surface.
2. Reinsch Test – Black deposit on copper strip.
3. Silver Nitrate Test – Yellow precipitate.
Arsine Gas (Garlic odour)
Black Deposit on Copper Strip
Yellow Precipitate
COMMON SOURCES
Pesticides, rat poisons, industrial effluents, contaminated water, some traditional medicines.
TOXIC EFFECTS (Key)
• Gastric irritation, vomiting, diarrhoea
• Burning pain in abdomen
• Peripheral neuropathy, skin lesions
• Carcinogenic in long term exposure
2. COPPER (Cu)
COPPER SULPHATE $CuSO_4$
IDENTIFICATION FEATURES
• Reddish-brown metal
• Forms bluish green salts (e.g., $CuSO_4$)
• Characteristic metallic taste (not safe to taste in lab)
• Soluble in acids
SIMPLE LAB IDENTIFICATION TESTS
1. With Ammonia – Deep blue solution.
2. With Potassium Ferrocyanide – Reddish brown precipitate.
3. Flame Test – Bluish green flame.
Deep Blue Solution (with NH_3)
Reddish Brown Precipitate
Bluish Green Flame
COMMON SOURCES
Copper utensils, fungicides, industrial waste, corroded pipes, contaminated water.
TOXIC EFFECTS (Key)
• Nausea, vomiting, abdominal pain
• Liver & kidney damage
• Hemolysis, jaundice
• Wilsonian effects in chronic exposure
3. MERCURY (Hg)
MERCURY Hg
IDENTIFICATION FEATURES
• Silvery, heavy liquid metal (only metal liquid at room temp.)
• Odourless
• Forms amalgam with other metals
• Common forms: Metallic Mercury, Mercuric chloride, Mercuric oxide (red)
SIMPLE LAB IDENTIFICATION TESTS
1. With Copper – Amalgam formation.
2. With Stannous Chloride – Gray/black precipitate.
3. Spot Test (for Hg^{2+}) – Black stain with Hg on filter paper by dipping in $SnCl_2$ solution.
Amalgam with Copper
Gray / Black Precipitate
Black Spot on Filter Paper
COMMON SOURCES
Thermometers, dental fillings, electrical switches, batteries, pesticides, cosmetics.
TOXIC EFFECTS (Key)
• Tremors, irritability, memory loss
• Gingivitis, hypersalivation
• Kidney damage
• Fetotoxic and neurotoxic
4. LEAD (Pb)
LEAD ACETATE $Pb(CH_3COO)_2$
IDENTIFICATION FEATURES
• Bluish-grey soft metal
• Malleable and heavy
• Forms soluble salts (e.g., Lead acetate)
• Insipid taste (DO NOT TASTE)
SIMPLE LAB IDENTIFICATION TESTS
1. With Potassium Iodide – Yellow precipitate (PbI_2).
2. With Sulphuric Acid – White precipitate ($PbSO_4$).
3. With Sodium Sulphide – Black precipitate (PbS).
Yellow Precipitate (PbI_2)
White Precipitate ($PbSO_4$)
Black Precipitate (PbS)
COMMON SOURCES
Paints, batteries, plumbing pipes, solder, industrial emissions, contaminated soil & water.
TOXIC EFFECTS (Key)
• Abdominal colic, constipation
• Anaemia (lead line in gums)
• Neuropathy, kidney damage
• Cognitive impairment in children
GENERAL PRECAUTIONS
Use Gloves & Mask
Work in Ventilated Area
Do Not Ingest or Inhale
Proper Waste Disposal
IDENTIFY – UNDERSTAND – PROTECT
Correct identification of toxic metals is crucial in diagnosis, treatment and prevention of poisoning.
Knowledge is the best antidote.
AGADA TANTRA PERSPECTIVE
✓ Visha is to be identified by its Rupa, Guna, Karma and Lakshana.
✓ Know the source, nature and effect of Visha for proper management.
✓ Agada (antidotes) and Shodhana (detoxification) save lives.
AGADA TANTRA
© COPYRIGHTS VISHA VAIDYA
Visha Vaidya
Dr Anil Kumar Y
Assistant Professor
Department of Agadatantra

PRACTICAL NO. 7

STHAVARA VISHA RECORD

Poisonous Plant	Botanical Name	Toxic Principle	Symptoms	Management
1.Dhattura				
2.Tobacco				
3.Gunja				
4.Karaveera				
5.Snuhi				
6.Jayapala				
7.Bhang				
8.Vatsanabha				

Poisonous Plant	Botanical Name	Toxic Principle	Symptoms	Management
9.Arka				
10.Langali				

Faculty Signature

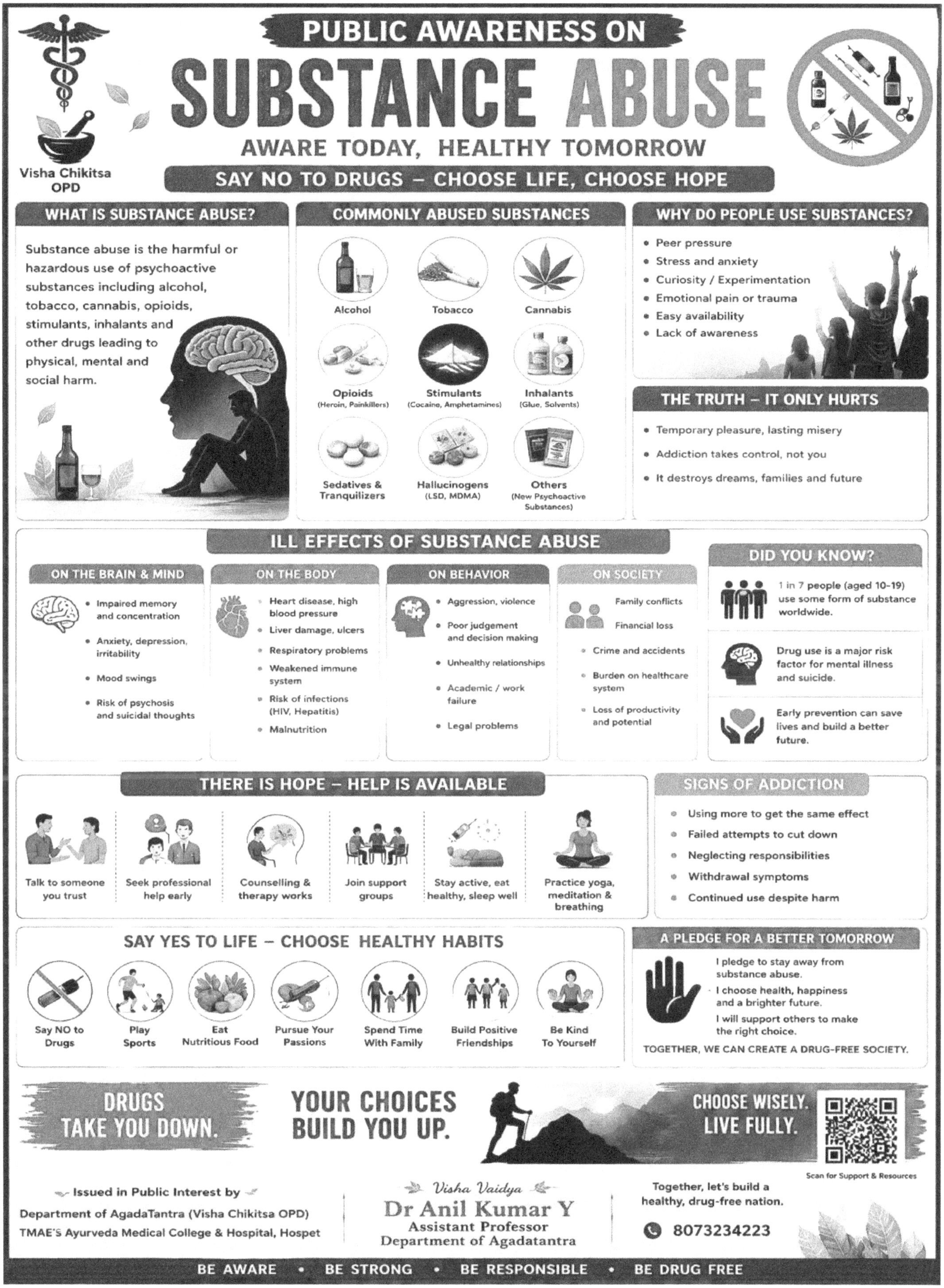
Visha Chikitsa OPD
PUBLIC AWARENESS ON
SUBSTANCE ABUSE
AWARE TODAY, HEALTHY TOMORROW
SAY NO TO DRUGS – CHOOSE LIFE, CHOOSE HOPE
WHAT IS SUBSTANCE ABUSE?
Substance abuse is the harmful or hazardous use of psychoactive substances including alcohol, tobacco, cannabis, opioids, stimulants, inhalants and other drugs leading to physical, mental and social harm.
COMMONLY ABUSED SUBSTANCES
Alcohol
Tobacco
Cannabis
Opioids (Heroin, Painkillers)
Stimulants (Cocaine, Amphetamines)
Inhalants (Glue, Solvents)
Sedatives & Tranquilizers
Hallucinogens (LSD, MDMA)
Others (New Psychoactive Substances)
WHY DO PEOPLE USE SUBSTANCES?
Peer pressure
Stress and anxiety
Curiosity / Experimentation
Emotional pain or trauma
Easy availability
Lack of awareness
THE TRUTH – IT ONLY HURTS
Temporary pleasure, lasting misery
Addiction takes control, not you
It destroys dreams, families and future
ILL EFFECTS OF SUBSTANCE ABUSE
ON THE BRAIN & MIND
Impaired memory and concentration
Anxiety, depression, irritability
Mood swings
Risk of psychosis and suicidal thoughts
ON THE BODY
Heart disease, high blood pressure
Liver damage, ulcers
Respiratory problems
Weakened immune system
Risk of infections (HIV, Hepatitis)
Malnutrition
ON BEHAVIOR
Aggression, violence
Poor judgement and decision making
Unhealthy relationships
Academic / work failure
Legal problems
ON SOCIETY
Family conflicts
Financial loss
Crime and accidents
Burden on healthcare system
Loss of productivity and potential
DID YOU KNOW?
1 in 7 people (aged 10-19) use some form of substance worldwide.
Drug use is a major risk factor for mental illness and suicide.
Early prevention can save lives and build a better future.
THERE IS HOPE – HELP IS AVAILABLE
Talk to someone you trust
Seek professional help early
Counselling & therapy works
Join support groups
Stay active, eat healthy, sleep well
Practice yoga, meditation & breathing
SIGNS OF ADDICTION
Using more to get the same effect
Failed attempts to cut down
Neglecting responsibilities
Withdrawal symptoms
Continued use despite harm
SAY YES TO LIFE – CHOOSE HEALTHY HABITS
Say NO to Drugs
Play Sports
Eat Nutritious Food
Pursue Your Passions
Spend Time With Family
Build Positive Friendships
Be Kind To Yourself
A PLEDGE FOR A BETTER TOMORROW
I pledge to stay away from substance abuse.
I choose health, happiness and a brighter future.
I will support others to make the right choice.
TOGETHER, WE CAN CREATE A DRUG-FREE SOCIETY.
DRUGS TAKE YOU DOWN.
YOUR CHOICES BUILD YOU UP.
CHOOSE WISELY. LIVE FULLY.
Scan for Support & Resources
Issued in Public Interest by
Department of AgadaTantra (Visha Chikitsa OPD)
TMAE's Ayurveda Medical College & Hospital, Hospet
Visha Vaidya
Dr Anil Kumar Y
Assistant Professor
Department of Agadatantra
Together, let's build a healthy, drug-free nation.
8073234223
BE AWARE • BE STRONG • BE RESPONSIBLE • BE DRUG FREE

PRACTICAL NO. 8

SUBSTANCE ABUSE CASE RECORD

Alcohol poisoning

Case No:01

Date:

Patient Details

Name::

Age::

Sex:

Address:

Occupation:

Chief Complaints:

History of Present Illness:

Duration of Addiction:

Exposure History:

Nidana:

Examination:

Samprapti:

Differential Diagnosis:

Diagnosis:

Treatment Given

Counselling:

Outcome

Discussion

Faculty Signature

PRACTICAL NO. 8

SUBSTANCE ABUSE CASE RECORD

Tobacco poisoning

Case No:02

Date:

Patient Details

Name::

Age::

Sex:

Address:

Occupation:

Chief Complaints:

History of Present Illness:

Duration of Addiction:

Exposure History:

Nidana:

Examination:

Samprapti:

Differential Diagnosis:

Diagnosis:

Treatment Given

Counselling:

Outcome

Discussion

Faculty Signature

PRACTICAL NO. 8

SUBSTANCE ABUSE CASE RECORD

Opioids/cannabis/other poisoning

Case No:04

Date:

Patient Details

Name::

Age::

Sex:

Address:

Occupation:

Chief Complaints:

History of Present Illness:

Duration of Addiction:

Exposure History:

Nidana:

Examination:

Samprapti:

Differential Diagnosis:

Diagnosis:

Treatment Given

Counselling:

Outcome

Discussion

Faculty Signature

Visha Chikitsa OPD

DEMONSTRATION ON
ISSUING OF FITNESS CERTIFICATE
RECENT ADVANCES IN NCISM & SUPREME COURT

JUSTICE • ETHICS • SERVICE

KNOW THE PROCESS – FOLLOW THE LAW – ENSURE JUSTICE

1. WHAT IS A FITNESS CERTIFICATE?

A Fitness Certificate is a medico-legal document issued by a Registered Medical Practitioner/Medical Board stating that a person is physically and mentally fit for a specific purpose.

FIT

2. WHEN IS A FITNESS CERTIFICATE REQUIRED?

- ✔ For employment (Govt./Private)
- ✔ For higher studies / admissions
- ✔ For marriage registration
- ✔ For driving license
- ✔ For travel (pilgrimage, sports, etc.)
- ✔ For insurance / military / police
- ✔ For any other legal requirement

3. ESSENTIAL COMPONENTS

- Patient's identification details
- Purpose of the certificate
- History and examination findings
- General physical fitness
- Mental fitness (if required)
- Investigations (if any)
- Opinion with date & signature
- Registration number & seal

4. FORMAT OF FITNESS CERTIFICATE (EXAMPLE)

Reg. No.: ____________ Date: ___/___/_____

FITNESS CERTIFICATE

This is to certify that I have examined

Mr./Ms. ______________________________

Age ______ Years, S/o / D/o ______________________

Residing at ______________________________

for the purpose of ______________________

and I am of the opinion that he / she is

PHYSICALLY AND MENTALLY FIT

for the above mentioned purpose.

Signature

Name: ______________

Qualification: ______________

Registration No.: ______________

Seal

REGISTERED MEDICAL PRACTITIONER

Note: The certificate should be genuine, truthful, objective and based on proper examination.

5. GUIDELINES FOR ISSUING

- ✔ Take proper history & do clinical examination
- ✔ Issue certificate only after satisfactory assessment
- ✔ Do not issue if unfit or information is insufficient
- ✔ Maintain confidentiality
- ✔ Keep medico-legal records safely
- ✔ Use official letterhead and seal
- ✔ Avoid overwriting and unauthorized alterations

6. LEGAL & ETHICAL RESPONSIBILITIES

- Issuing a false certificate is a punishable offence under IPC & MCI/NCISM regulations
- You are legally accountable for every certificate issued
- Act with honesty, integrity and professional ethics
- "Do No Harm" includes "Do No Wrong"

7. RECENT ADVANCES IN NCISM (National Commission for Indian System of Medicine)

Outcome Based Education (OBE)
Competency based curriculum with clear learning outcomes.

Integrated Medical Education
Integration of Ayurveda with modern medical science & research.

Assessment Reforms
Standardized assessment pattern, AETCOM, OSCE, & formative assessments.

Research & Innovation
Emphasis on evidence based research and innovation in AYUSH systems.

Digital Initiatives
e-Samiksha, digital portals, online attachments, & academic automation.

Faculty Development
Capacity building programs, workshops, and continuous professional development.

NCISM Vision: Quality Education – Ethical Practice – Research Excellence – Holistic Healthcare

8. RECENT SUPREME COURT JUDGEMENTS – KEY HIGHLIGHTS (Relevant to Medical Professionals)

Professional Negligence
- Doctors must follow standard protocols and act with reasonable care.
- Negligence leading to harm = Legal Liability.

Informed Consent
- Informed consent is mandatory.
- Non-disclosure of risk is professional misconduct.

Documentation is Crucial
- Proper records are your best defence.
- Poor documentation leads to presumption of negligence.

Respect for Patient Rights
- Patient autonomy and dignity must be respected.
- Right to information is a fundamental right.

Consumer Protection Act Applicable
- Medical services come under Consumer Protection Act.
- Patients can file complaints.

Good Samaritan Protection
- Good Samaritan guidelines are protected.
- Doctors helping in emergencies are legally safeguarded.

9. DOCTORS – YOUR DUTY

- ✔ Be Competent
- ✔ Be Compassionate
- ✔ Be Ethical
- ✔ Be Honest
- ✔ Be Updated
- ✔ Be Accountable

10. PROCESS FLOW – ISSUING FITNESS CERTIFICATE

Take History → Clinical Examination → Investigations (If required) → Evaluate Fitness → Issue Certificate with Seal & Sign → Maintain Record

11. REMEMBER

"A Certificate is not just a paper, it is a reflection of your ethics, knowledge & responsibility."

For More Awareness Scan QR Code

Visha Vaidya
Dr Anil Kumar Y
Assistant Professor
Department of Agada Tantra (Visha Chikitsa OPD)
TMAE's Ayurveda Medical College & Hospital, Hospet

"Right Certificate, Right Person, Right Purpose, Right Future."

PRACTICAL NO. 9

LEGAL PROCEDURES

Medico-Legal Case Report Format

EMERGENCY POLICE INTIMATION

Date: ___________ Time: ___________

To,
SHO,
________________ Police Station

Sir/Madam,

A **medico-legal case has been admitted in our hospital.

Patient Name: ____________________
Age/Sex: ________________________
MLC No.: ________________________
Date & Time of Admission: _________

Alleged History:

Present Condition:

This is for necessary legal action.

Medical Officer
(Signature & Seal)

MLC No:

** Cases Requiring Immediate Police Intimation

- Road Traffic Accidents (RTA)
- Assault and injuries
- Poisoning (suicidal, accidental, homicidal)
- Burns (especially >20% or suspicious burns)
- Snakebite with suspicious circumstances
- Firearm injuries
- Sexual offences
- Attempted suicide
- Electrocution
- Unknown or unconscious patients
- Death on arrival (DOA)
- Custodial injuries

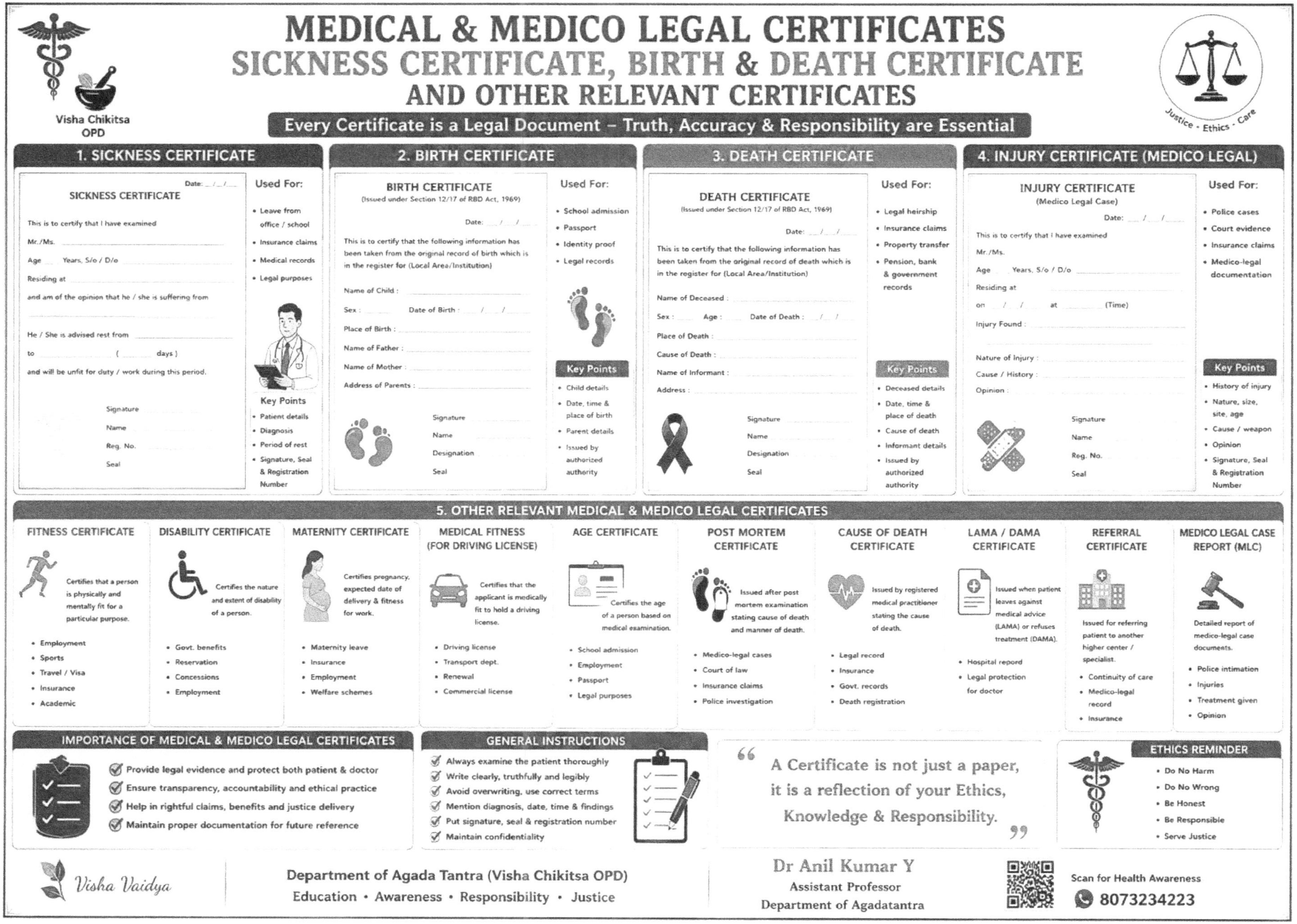
Visha Chikitsa OPD
MEDICAL & MEDICO LEGAL CERTIFICATES
SICKNESS CERTIFICATE, BIRTH & DEATH CERTIFICATE
AND OTHER RELEVANT CERTIFICATES
Every Certificate is a Legal Document – Truth, Accuracy & Responsibility are Essential
Justice · Ethics · Care
1. SICKNESS CERTIFICATE
SICKNESS CERTIFICATE
Date: __/__/__
This is to certify that I have examined
Mr./Ms.
Age Years, S/o / D/o
Residing at
and am of the opinion that he / she is suffering from
He / She is advised rest from
to (days)
and will be unfit for duty / work during this period.
Signature
Name
Reg. No.
Seal
Used For:
• Leave from office / school
• Insurance claims
• Medical records
• Legal purposes
Key Points
• Patient details
• Diagnosis
• Period of rest
• Signature, Seal & Registration Number
2. BIRTH CERTIFICATE
BIRTH CERTIFICATE
(Issued under Section 12/17 of RBD Act, 1969)
Date: __/__/__
This is to certify that the following information has been taken from the original record of birth which is in the register for (Local Area/Institution)
Name of Child :
Sex : Date of Birth : / /
Place of Birth :
Name of Father :
Name of Mother :
Address of Parents :
Signature
Name
Designation
Seal
Used For:
• School admission
• Passport
• Identity proof
• Legal records
Key Points
• Child details
• Date, time & place of birth
• Parent details
• Issued by authorized authority
3. DEATH CERTIFICATE
DEATH CERTIFICATE
(Issued under Section 12/17 of RBD Act, 1969)
Date: __/__/__
This is to certify that the following information has been taken from the original record of death which is in the register for (Local Area/Institution)
Name of Deceased :
Sex : Age : Date of Death : / /
Place of Death :
Cause of Death :
Name of Informant :
Address :
Signature
Name
Designation
Seal
Used For:
• Legal heirship
• Insurance claims
• Property transfer
• Pension, bank & government records
Key Points
• Deceased details
• Date, time & place of death
• Cause of death
• Informant details
• Issued by authorized authority
4. INJURY CERTIFICATE (MEDICO LEGAL)
INJURY CERTIFICATE
(Medico Legal Case)
Date: __/__/__
This is to certify that I have examined
Mr./Ms.
Age Years, S/o / D/o
Residing at
on / / at (Time)
Injury Found :
Nature of Injury :
Cause / History :
Opinion :
Signature
Name
Reg. No.
Seal
Used For:
• Police cases
• Court evidence
• Insurance claims
• Medico-legal documentation
Key Points
• History of injury
• Nature, size, site, age
• Cause / weapon
• Opinion
• Signature, Seal & Registration Number
5. OTHER RELEVANT MEDICAL & MEDICO LEGAL CERTIFICATES
FITNESS CERTIFICATE
Certifies that a person is physically and mentally fit for a particular purpose.
• Employment
• Sports
• Travel / Visa
• Insurance
• Academic
DISABILITY CERTIFICATE
Certifies the nature and extent of disability of a person.
• Govt. benefits
• Reservation
• Concessions
• Employment
MATERNITY CERTIFICATE
Certifies pregnancy, expected date of delivery & fitness for work.
• Maternity leave
• Insurance
• Employment
• Welfare schemes
MEDICAL FITNESS (FOR DRIVING LICENSE)
Certifies that the applicant is medically fit to hold a driving license.
• Driving license
• Transport dept.
• Renewal
• Commercial license
AGE CERTIFICATE
Certifies the age of a person based on medical examination.
• School admission
• Employment
• Passport
• Legal purposes
POST MORTEM CERTIFICATE
Issued after post mortem examination stating cause of death and manner of death.
• Medico-legal cases
• Court of law
• Insurance claims
• Police investigation
CAUSE OF DEATH CERTIFICATE
Issued by registered medical practitioner stating the cause of death.
• Legal record
• Insurance
• Govt. records
• Death registration
LAMA / DAMA CERTIFICATE
Issued when patient leaves against medical advice (LAMA) or refuses treatment (DAMA).
• Hospital record
• Legal protection for doctor
REFERRAL CERTIFICATE
Issued for referring patient to another higher center / specialist.
• Continuity of care
• Medico-legal record
• Insurance
MEDICO LEGAL CASE REPORT (MLC)
Detailed report of medico-legal case documents.
• Police intimation
• Injuries
• Treatment given
• Opinion
IMPORTANCE OF MEDICAL & MEDICO LEGAL CERTIFICATES
Provide legal evidence and protect both patient & doctor
Ensure transparency, accountability and ethical practice
Help in rightful claims, benefits and justice delivery
Maintain proper documentation for future reference
GENERAL INSTRUCTIONS
Always examine the patient thoroughly
Write clearly, truthfully and legibly
Avoid overwriting, use correct terms
Mention diagnosis, date, time & findings
Put signature, seal & registration number
Maintain confidentiality
“A Certificate is not just a paper, it is a reflection of your Ethics, Knowledge & Responsibility.”
ETHICS REMINDER
• Do No Harm
• Do No Wrong
• Be Honest
• Be Responsible
• Serve Justice
Visha Vaidya
Department of Agada Tantra (Visha Chikitsa OPD)
Education • Awareness • Responsibility • Justice
Dr Anil Kumar Y
Assistant Professor
Department of Agadatantra
Scan for Health Awareness
8073234223

PRACTICAL NO. 9

LEGAL PROCEDURES

MEDICAL FITNESS CERTIFICATE

Name of Hospital/Clinic
Address: ________________________________
Phone: _________________________________

Certificate No.: ________________________
Date: __________________________________

TO WHOMSOEVER IT MAY CONCERN

This is to certify that I have medically examined
Mr./Ms.____________________________________,

Age: ___________ Years
Sex: ___________
Address: ____

The individual was examined on _____________ (date) and was found to be in satisfactory physical and mental health.

At the time of examination:

- General Condition: Good
- Pulse Rate: __________ per minute
- Blood Pressure: __________ mmHg
- Respiratory System: Normal
- Cardiovascular System: Normal
- Central Nervous System: Normal
- Locomotor System: Normal
- Vision: Normal / Corrected
- Hearing: Normal

In my opinion, the above-mentioned individual is medically fit to perform duties/studies/travel/sports activities as required.

Purpose of Certificate:

This certificate is issued on the request of the individual for the above-mentioned purpose.

Signature of Medical Officer

Name: ________________________________
Qualification: __________________________
Registration No.: _______________________
Hospital/Clinic Seal

FITNESS CERTIFICATE AFTER ILLNESS

Date: ___________________

This is to certify that Mr./Ms. _____________________________,
Age ______ years, was under my treatment for
_______________________________ from __________ to __________.

The patient has recovered satisfactorily and is medically fit to resume duties/work/studies with effect from _____________.

Doctor's Signature
Name:
Qualification:
Registration No.:
Seal

PRACTICAL NO. 9

LEGAL PROCEDURES

SICKNESS CERTIFICATE

Name of Hospital/Clinic
Address: ______________________________

Certificate No.: ______________________
Date: ______________________________

TO WHOMSOEVER IT MAY CONCERN

This is to certify that I have examined Mr./Ms.
______________________________________,

Age: _______ Years
Sex: _______
Address: ____

The patient is suffering from
____.

Due to the above illness, the patient has been advised complete rest and is medically unfit to attend duties/work/classes from _____________ to _____________.

The patient is expected to resume normal activities after recovery and medical reassessment, if required.

This certificate is issued on the basis of clinical examination and at the request of the patient for official purposes.

Place: ____________________

Date: _____________________

Signature of Medical Officer

Name: ______________________________
Qualification: _____________________
Registration No.: __________________
Hospital/Clinic Seal

PRACTICAL NO. 9

LEGAL PROCEDURES

MEDICAL CERTIFICATE OF BIRTH

Hospital Name: ______________________________
Address: ___________________________________

Certificate No.: ___________________________
Date of Issue: _____________________________

1. Details of Child

Name of Child (if given): _________________________

Sex:
□ Male
□ Female
□ Other

Date of Birth: ______________________________

Time of Birth: ______________________________

Place of Birth:

Type of Birth:
□ Single
□ Twin
□ Multiple

Birth Weight: ____________ kg

2. Details of Mother

Name of Mother:

Age: ___________ Years

Address:

Hospital Registration Number:

3. Details of Father

Name of Father:

Age: __________ Years

Address (if different):

4. Certification

This is to certify that the above-mentioned child was born in this hospital/institution on the date and time stated above.

Place: ________________________________

Date: ________________________________

Signature of Attending Doctor

Name: ________________________________

Qualification: ___________________________

Registration No.: _________________________

Hospital Seal

BIRTH CERTIFICATE

This is to certify that a live child was born to Mrs.

____

wife of Mr. ________________________________

on ______________ (date) at ______________ (time)

at ____ Hospital.

Sex of Child: ______________________________

Birth Weight: ______________________________

Doctor's Signature
Name:
Registration No.:
Hospital Seal

PRACTICAL NO. 9

LEGAL PROCEDURES

MEDICAL CERTIFICATE OF CAUSE OF DEATH

Hospital Name: ___________________________
Address: ________________________________

Certificate No.: _________________________

1. Particulars of Deceased

Name: ________________________________

Age/Sex: ______________________________

Address: ______________________________

Hospital Registration No.: ______________

Date of Admission: ______________________

Date and Time of Death: _________________

2. Cause of Death

Immediate Cause:

Due to (Antecedent Cause):

Due to (Underlying Cause):

Other Significant Conditions Contributing to Death:

Approximate Interval Between Onset and Death:

3. Certification

I hereby certify that I attended the deceased during the last illness and, to the best of my knowledge and belief, the above-mentioned cause of death is correct.

Place: ______________________________

Date: ______________________________

Signature of Medical Officer

Name: ______________________________

Qualification: ______________________

Registration No.: ____________________

Hospital Seal

Visha Chikitsa OPD

DEMONSTRATION OF REPORTING OF LAMA, DAMA & DOPR

MEDICO LEGAL DOCUMENTATION

• LEAVE AGAINST MEDICAL ADVICE • DISCHARGE AGAINST MEDICAL ADVICE • DISCHARGE ON PATIENT REQUEST

INFORM – DOCUMENT – COUNSEL – RESPECT – RECORD

1. LAMA – LEAVE AGAINST MEDICAL ADVICE

When a patient, who is advised hospitalization or treatment, decides to leave the hospital against the medical advice of the treating doctor.

LAMA REPORT (Format)

Name of Patient : ______
Age / Sex : ____ / ____ UHID / IP No. : ______
Date & Time of Admission : ______
Date & Time of LAMA : ______
Provisional Diagnosis : ______
Treatment / Advice Given : ______

I, Dr. ______ have explained to the patient / attendant in detail about the illness, necessary investigations, treatment, risks of leaving the hospital, possible complications including death.

Despite explaining, the patient / attendant is leaving the hospital against medical advice.

Patient / Attendant Name : ______
Relation with Patient : ______
Signature / Thumb Impression : ______
Date & Time : ______
Name & Signature of Doctor : ______
Designation ______
Witness Name & Signature (Staff / Relative) : ______

Note: LAMA is not recommended. Patient is informed about the consequences and responsibility.

2. DAMA – DISCHARGE AGAINST MEDICAL ADVICE

When a patient, who is admitted and under treatment, discontinues treatment and requests for discharge against medical advice.

DAMA REPORT (Format)

Name of Patient : ______
Age / Sex : ____ / ____ UHID / IP No. : ______
Date & Time of Admission : ______
Date & Time of DAMA : ______
Diagnosis : ______
Summary of Treatment Given : ______

I, Dr. ______ have explained to the patient / attendant about the condition, treatment plan, possible complications and risks of discontinuing treatment.

Despite explaining, the patient / attendant insists on discharge against medical advice.

Patient / Attendant Name : ______
Relation with Patient : ______
Reason for DAMA (as stated by patient/attendant): ______

Signature / Thumb Impression : ______
Date & Time : ______
Name & Signature of Doctor : ______
Designation : ______
Witness Name & Signature (Staff / Relative) : ______

Note: Patient is aware of the risks and takes full responsibility.

3. DOPR – DISCHARGE ON PATIENT REQUEST

When a patient who is stable / fit for discharge requests for discharge after completing treatment or against further continuation.

DOPR REPORT (Format)

Name of Patient : ______
Age / Sex : ____ / ____ UHID / IP No. : ______
Date & Time of Admission : ______
Date & Time of Discharge : ______
Diagnosis : ______
Treatment Given : ______

I, Dr. ______ certify that patient is currently stable / fit for discharge and the patient / attendant has requested for discharge.

Patient / Attendant Name : ______
Relation with Patient : ______
Patient Condition on Discharge : Stable / Improved / Recovered
Advice on Discharge : ______

Signature / Thumb Impression : ______
Date & Time : ______
Name & Signature of Doctor : ______
Designation : ______
Witness Name & Signature (Staff / Relative) : ______

Note: Patient discharged as per request and informed advice given.

KEY POINTS TO REMEMBER

- Always explain the diagnosis, treatment, risks & consequences.
- Inform in simple language and ensure patient / attendant understands.
- Document the explanation clearly.
- Take signature/thumb impression of patient / attendant.
- Make an entry in case sheet and hospital register.
- Inform concerned authority if needed.

GENERAL INSTRUCTIONS

- Counsel the patient to continue treatment.
- Encourage patient to follow medical advice.
- Respect patient's decision after proper explanation.
- Maintain proper documentation for medico-legal safety.
- Ensure witness signature (staff/relative).

IMPORTANCE OF PROPER REPORTING

- Protects patient's rights & safety.
- Protects doctor/hospital in legal matters.
- Ensures transparency & ethical practice.
- Essential for quality healthcare & accountability.

DOCUMENT TODAY, PROTECT TOMORROW

Visha Vaidya
Dr Anil Kumar Y
Assistant Professor
Department of Agada Tantra (Visha Chikitsa OPD)
TMAE's Ayurveda Medical College & Hospital, Hospet

"Good Documentation is Good Medical Practice and Good Legal Protection."

Scan for Health Awareness & Patient Education
8073234223

PRACTICAL NO. 9

LEGAL PROCEDURES

DEATH CONFIRMATION CERTIFICATE

This is to certify that Mr./Mrs. ____________________________,
Age ______ years, was examined by me and was found to have expired on
_____________ at _____________ hours.

On examination, the following signs of death were observed:

- Absence of pulse
- Absence of heart sounds
- Absence of respiration
- Fixed and dilated pupils

The death was confirmed at _____________ hours on _____________.

Doctor's Signature
Name:
Registration No.:
Hospital Seal

Important Medico-Legal Note

Police intimation is mandatory before issuing a death certificate in cases such as:

- Road traffic accidents
- Poisoning
- Burns
- Hanging
- Drowning
- Electrocution
- Firearm injuries
- Assault
- Sudden unexplained deaths
- Deaths in custody
- Any suspicious or unnatural death

These cases require medico-legal investigation and usually post-mortem examination before the final cause of death is established.

PRACTICAL NO. 9

LEGAL PROCEDURES

LEAVE AGAINST MEDICAL ADVICE (LAMA) REPORT

Hospital Name: ____________________________
Department: ______________________________

LAMA No.: _______________________________
Date: ________________ Time: ______________

Patient Details

Name: _________________________________

Age/Sex: _______________________________

Address: _______________________________

Hospital Registration No.: _______________

Date of Admission: ______________________

Diagnosis/Provisional Diagnosis:

Present Condition of Patient:

I, Mr./Ms./Mrs. ___________________________
(Patient/Relative/Guardian), have been informed by the treating doctor regarding:

- The nature of the illness/injury.
- The need for further investigations and treatment.
- The possible risks and complications of discontinuing treatment.
- The possibility of worsening of the condition, permanent disability, or death.

Despite understanding the above information, I wish to leave the hospital against medical advice and on my own responsibility.

Reason for LAMA:

The hospital authorities and treating doctors shall not be held responsible for any adverse consequences resulting from my decision to leave against medical advice.

Patient/Guardian Signature/Thumb Impression:

Name of Patient/Guardian:

Relationship (if guardian):

Witness 1:
Name & Signature:

Witness 2:
Name & Signature:

Treating Doctor's Certification

I have explained the patient's condition, treatment plan, and possible consequences of leaving the hospital against medical advice.

Doctor's Signature:

Name:

Designation:

Registration No.:

Hospital Seal

PRACTICAL NO. 9

LEGAL PROCEDURES

DISCHARGE AGAINST MEDICAL ADVICE (DAMA)

Hospital Name: ______________________________
Department/Ward: ___________________________

DAMA No.: __________________________________
Date: _______________ Time: _______________

PATIENT DETAILS

Name: ____________________________________

Age/Sex: __________________________________

IP No.: ___________________________________

Address: __________________________________

Date of Admission: ______________________

Provisional/Final Diagnosis:

Present Clinical Condition:

Treating Doctor's Advice:

DECLARATION BY PATIENT/GUARDIAN

I, Mr./Ms./Mrs. ____________________________,
the patient/legal guardian of the above patient, have been informed in a language understood by me regarding:

1. The patient's diagnosis and present condition.
2. The need for continued hospitalization and treatment.
3. The risks of discontinuing treatment.
4. Possible complications including deterioration of health, permanent disability, or death.

Despite understanding the above information, I voluntarily request discharge against medical advice and take full responsibility for this decision.

Reason for DAMA:

I release the hospital and treating doctors from responsibility for adverse outcomes resulting from my decision.

Patient/Guardian Signature:

Name:

Relationship (if guardian):

Date & Time:

WITNESSES

1. Name & Signature:

2. Name & Signature:

CERTIFICATION BY TREATING DOCTOR

I have explained the patient's condition, treatment requirements, prognosis, and possible risks of leaving the hospital against medical advice. The patient/guardian has understood the explanation and still wishes to leave.

Doctor's Signature:

Name:

Designation:

Registration No.:

Hospital Seal

PRACTICAL NO. 9

LEGAL PROCEDURES

DISCHARGE ON PATIENT REQUEST (DOPR)

Hospital Name: ____________________________
Department/Ward: __________________________

DOPR No.: ________________________________
Date: ______________ Time: ______________

PATIENT DETAILS

Name: ________________________________

Age/Sex: ______________________________

IP No.: _______________________________

Address: ______________________________

Date of Admission: ___________________________

Date of Discharge: ___________________________

Diagnosis:

Present Clinical Status:

DECLARATION BY PATIENT/GUARDIAN

I, Mr./Ms./Mrs. ____________________________,
request discharge from the hospital on my own request.

I have been informed about:

- My current medical condition.
- The treatment received during hospitalization.
- Further treatment/follow-up advice.
- Possible risks associated with discontinuation of inpatient care.

I understand the advice provided by the treating doctor and voluntarily request discharge from the hospital.

Reason for Request:

I undertake responsibility for compliance with the treatment and follow-up instructions provided.

Patient/Guardian Signature:

Name:

Relationship (if guardian):

Date & Time:

TREATING DOCTOR'S CERTIFICATE

The patient has requested discharge. The patient's present condition, treatment received, medications, and follow-up instructions have been explained. The patient/guardian has understood the advice and requested discharge.

Doctor's Signature:

Name:

Designation:

Registration No.:

NURSING OFFICER SIGNATURE

Name:

Signature:

Hospital Seal

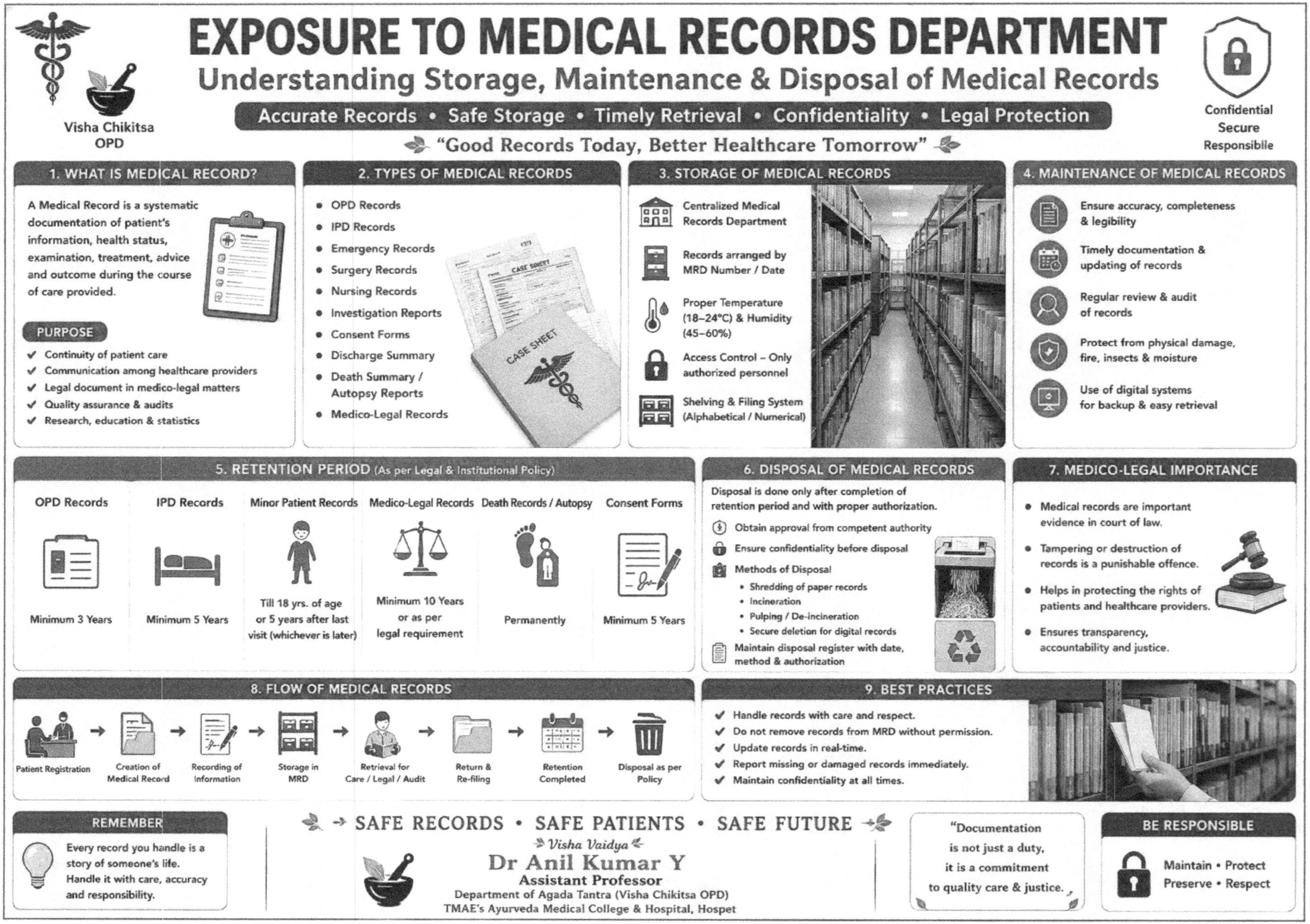

Visha Chikitsa OPD
EXPOSURE TO MEDICAL RECORDS DEPARTMENT
Understanding Storage, Maintenance & Disposal of Medical Records
Accurate Records • Safe Storage • Timely Retrieval • Confidentiality • Legal Protection
"Good Records Today, Better Healthcare Tomorrow"
Confidential
Secure
Responsibile
1. WHAT IS MEDICAL RECORD?
A Medical Record is a systematic documentation of patient's information, health status, examination, treatment, advice and outcome during the course of care provided.
PURPOSE
✔ Continuity of patient care
✔ Communication among healthcare providers
✔ Legal document in medico-legal matters
✔ Quality assurance & audits
✔ Research, education & statistics
2. TYPES OF MEDICAL RECORDS
• OPD Records
• IPD Records
• Emergency Records
• Surgery Records
• Nursing Records
• Investigation Reports
• Consent Forms
• Discharge Summary
• Death Summary / Autopsy Reports
• Medico-Legal Records
CASE SHEET
3. STORAGE OF MEDICAL RECORDS
Centralized Medical Records Department
Records arranged by MRD Number / Date
Proper Temperature (18–24°C) & Humidity (45–60%)
Access Control – Only authorized personnel
Shelving & Filing System (Alphabetical / Numerical)
4. MAINTENANCE OF MEDICAL RECORDS
Ensure accuracy, completeness & legibility
Timely documentation & updating of records
Regular review & audit of records
Protect from physical damage, fire, insects & moisture
Use of digital systems for backup & easy retrieval
5. RETENTION PERIOD (As per Legal & Institutional Policy)
OPD Records — Minimum 3 Years
IPD Records — Minimum 5 Years
Minor Patient Records — Till 18 yrs. of age or 5 years after last visit (whichever is later)
Medico-Legal Records — Minimum 10 Years or as per legal requirement
Death Records / Autopsy — Permanently
Consent Forms — Minimum 5 Years
6. DISPOSAL OF MEDICAL RECORDS
Disposal is done only after completion of retention period and with proper authorization.
Obtain approval from competent authority
Ensure confidentiality before disposal
Methods of Disposal
• Shredding of paper records
• Incineration
• Pulping / De-incineration
• Secure deletion for digital records
Maintain disposal register with date, method & authorization
7. MEDICO-LEGAL IMPORTANCE
• Medical records are important evidence in court of law.
• Tampering or destruction of records is a punishable offence.
• Helps in protecting the rights of patients and healthcare providers.
• Ensures transparency, accountability and justice.
8. FLOW OF MEDICAL RECORDS
Patient Registration → Creation of Medical Record → Recording of Information → Storage in MRD → Retrieval for Care / Legal / Audit → Return & Re-filing → Retention Completed → Disposal as per Policy
9. BEST PRACTICES
✔ Handle records with care and respect.
✔ Do not remove records from MRD without permission.
✔ Update records in real-time.
✔ Report missing or damaged records immediately.
✔ Maintain confidentiality at all times.
REMEMBER
Every record you handle is a story of someone's life. Handle it with care, accuracy and responsibility.
→ SAFE RECORDS • SAFE PATIENTS • SAFE FUTURE →
Visha Vaidya
Dr Anil Kumar Y
Assistant Professor
Department of Agada Tantra (Visha Chikitsa OPD)
TMAE's Ayurveda Medical College & Hospital, Hospet
"Documentation is not just a duty, it is a commitment to quality care & justice."
BE RESPONSIBLE
Maintain • Protect
Preserve • Respect

PRACTICAL NO. 10

VAIDYA SADVRITTA

EXPOSURE TO MEDICAL RECORDS DEPARTMENT (MRD)

Date : ___________

Title of Practical

Exposure to the Medical Records Department for Understanding the Storage, Maintenance and Disposal of Medical Records

Objectives

1. To observe the functioning of the Medical Records Department (MRD).
2. To understand the methods of storage and maintenance of medical records.
3. To study the retrieval and preservation of patient records.
4. To understand the retention and disposal procedures of medical records.

Observation

Sl. No.	Particulars Observed	Findings
1	Name of Hospital	____________________
2	Location of MRD	____________________
3	Type of Record System	Manual / Electronic / Hybrid
4	Records Maintained	OPD / IPD / MLC / Birth & Death Records
5	Method of Storage	Shelves / Compactors / Digital Storage
6	Record Numbering System	____________________
7	Coding System Used	ICD / Other
8	Record Retrieval Method	____________________
9	Confidentiality Measures	____________________
10	Record Retention Policy	____________________
11	Disposal Method	Shredding / Incineration / Digital Deletion

Sl. No.	Particulars Observed	Findings
12	Authority for Disposal	____________________

Procedure Observed

1. Registration of patient records.
2. Assignment of unique hospital number.
3. Filing and storage of records.
4. Coding and indexing of records.
5. Retrieval of records when required.
6. Preservation and retention as per hospital policy.
7. Disposal of records after completion of retention period.

Learning Points

- Medical records are important legal documents.
- Proper storage ensures easy retrieval and preservation.
- Confidentiality of patient information must be maintained.
- Disposal of records should be carried out according to institutional guidelines.

Result

Teacher's Signature

Student's Signature

Visha Chikitsa OPD

DEMONSTRATE THE METHOD OF
SEX DETERMINATION BASED ON PELVIS

THE PELVIS IS THE MOST RELIABLE PART OF THE SKELETON FOR SEX DETERMINATION IN ADULTS

Forensic Science For Justice

1. WHY PELVIS?

- ✓ The pelvis shows marked sexual dimorphism.
- ✓ It reflects reproductive function and hormonal influence.
- ✓ Highly reliable in adult skeleton.

DO NOT USE IN CHILDREN (before puberty)

2. MALE PELVIS – CHARACTERISTICS

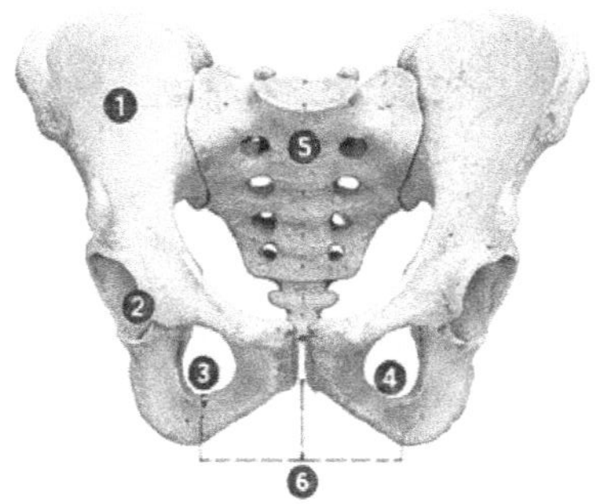

1. **Ilium**
   Less flared, relatively vertical
2. **Greater Sciatic Notch**
   Narrow and V-shaped
3. **Subpubic Angle (Pubic Arch)**
   Narrow (< 70°)
4. **Ischial Spines**
   Prominent, directed inwards
5. **Sacrum**
   Long, narrow, more curved
6. **Obturator Foramen**
   Oval, smaller

2. FEMALE PELVIS – CHARACTERISTICS

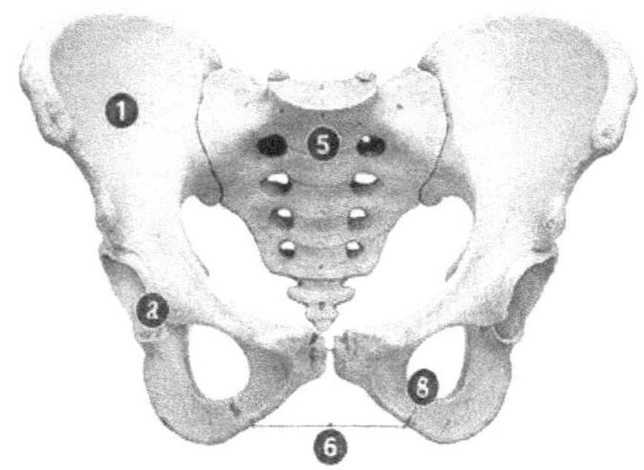

1. **Ilium**
   Wide, flared, laterally spread
2. **Greater Sciatic Notch**
   Wide and U-shaped
3. **Subpubic Angle (Pubic Arch)**
   Wide (> 80°), U-shaped
4. **Ischial Spines**
   Less prominent, everted
5. **Sacrum**
   Short, wide, less curved
6. **Obturator Foramen**
   Round/triangular, larger

3. SIDE VIEW COMPARISON

MALE PELVIS (LATERAL VIEW)

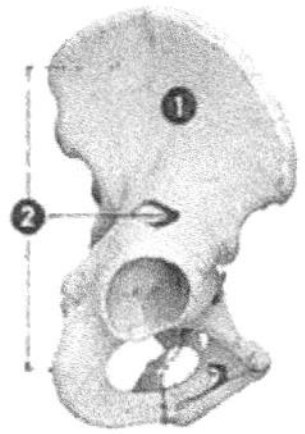

1. **Ilium**
   Relatively vertical
2. **Sacrum**
   Narrow, more curved
3. **Pubic Symphysis**
   Narrow and tall

FEMALE PELVIS (LATERAL VIEW)

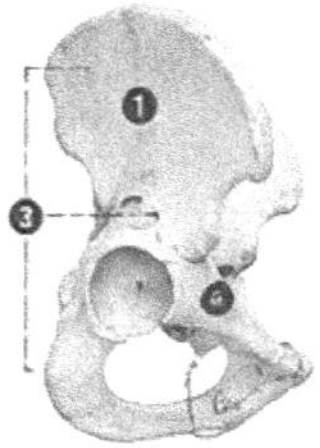

1. **Ilium**
   Well flared
2. **Sacrum**
   Wide, less curved
3. **Pubic Symphysis**
   Wide and short

4. SUBPUBIC ANGLE (PUBIC ARCH)

MALE
NARROW ANGLE
(< 70°)

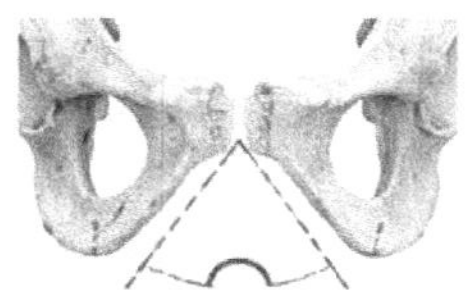

FEMALE
WIDE ANGLE
(> 80°)

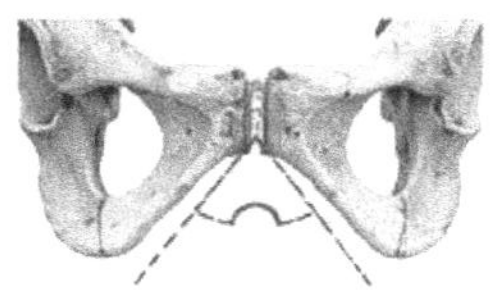

5. KEY DIFFERENCES AT A GLANCE

Feature	Male	Female
Ilium	Less flared	Wide and flared
Greater Sciatic Notch	Narrow (V-shaped)	Wide (U-shaped)
Subpubic Angle	Narrow (< 70°)	Wide (> 80°)
Ischial Spines	Prominent, inturned	Less prominent, everted
Sacrum	Long, narrow, more curved	Short, wide, less curved
Obturator Foramen	Oval, smaller	Round/triangular, larger
Pubic Symphysis	Narrow, tall	Wide, short

6. METHOD / STEPS

1. Clean the pelvis and observe overall size and robustness.
2. Observe the ilium – note the degree of flaring.
3. Examine the greater sciatic notch – note shape and width.
4. Measure the subpubic angle using a goniometer.
5. Observe ischial spines – note prominence and direction.
6. Observe sacrum – note length, width and curvature.
7. Examine obturator foramen – note shape and size.
8. Observe pubic symphysis – note height and width.
9. Consider all features together before giving opinion.

Note: No single feature should be used alone.

7. INSTRUMENTS REQUIRED

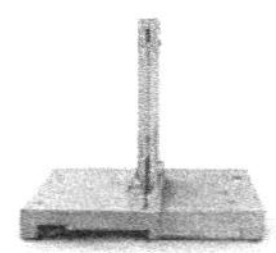

Osteometric Board

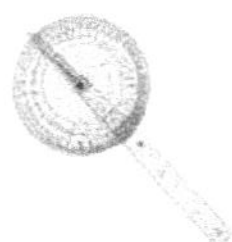

Goniometer

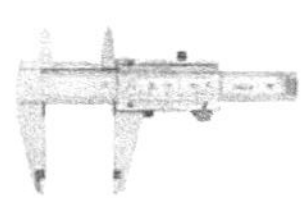

Sliding Caliper

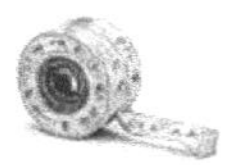

Measuring Tape

8. IMPORTANT POINTS

- ✓ Most reliable method in adult skeleton.
- ✓ Not reliable in fragmented or damaged pelvis.
- ✓ Consider all features collectively.
- ✓ Provide opinion as: Male / Female / Indeterminate.
- ✓ Report should mention reasons and features considered.

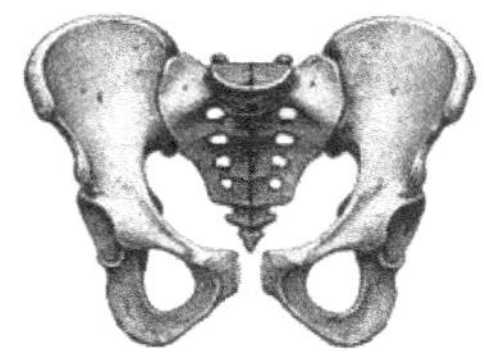

Scan for Study Material & Videos

Visha Vaidya

Dr Anil Kumar Y
Assistant Professor
Department of Agada Tantra (Visha Chikitsa OPD)
TMAE's Ayurveda Medical College & Hospital, Hospete

" Science seeks the truth, Forensics brings justice. "

Truth
Accuracy
Justice
Responsibility

PRACTICAL NO. 11

PERSONAL IDENTITY

SEX DETERMINATION BASED ON PELVIS

Date:

Aim

Materials Required

Principle

The pelvis is the most reliable bone for sex determination because it shows marked differences between males and females, mainly due to adaptation for childbirth.

Observations

Feature	Male Pelvis	Female Pelvis	Specimen Observed
General Build	Heavy and thick	Light and thin	__________
Pelvic Cavity	Narrow and deep	Wide and shallow	__________
Pelvic Inlet	Heart-shaped	Oval/Round	__________
Subpubic Angle	< 70° (Narrow)	> 80–90° (Wide)	__________
Greater Sciatic Notch	Narrow	Wide	__________
Sacrum	Long and curved	Short and broad	__________
Obturator Foramen	Large and oval	Small and triangular	__________
Ischial Spines	Project inward	Less prominent	__________

Key Identification Points

Male Pelvis

- Heavy and rugged
- Heart-shaped pelvic inlet
- Narrow subpubic angle
- Narrow sciatic notch
- Deep pelvic cavity

Female Pelvis

- Light and smooth
- Oval/round pelvic inlet
- Wide subpubic angle
- Wide sciatic notch
- Broad pelvic cavity

FEMALE = "WOMB"

- **W** = Wide sciatic notch
- **O** = Oval pelvic inlet
- **M** = More subpubic angle (>90°)
- **B** = Broad pelvis

MALE = "HEART"

- **H** = Heart-shaped inlet
- **E** = Extended deep cavity
- **A** = Acute subpubic angle
- **R** = Rugged/heavy bone
- **T** = Tight (narrow) sciatic notch

Result

Conclusion

Teacher's Signature: ____________________

Student's Signature: ____________________

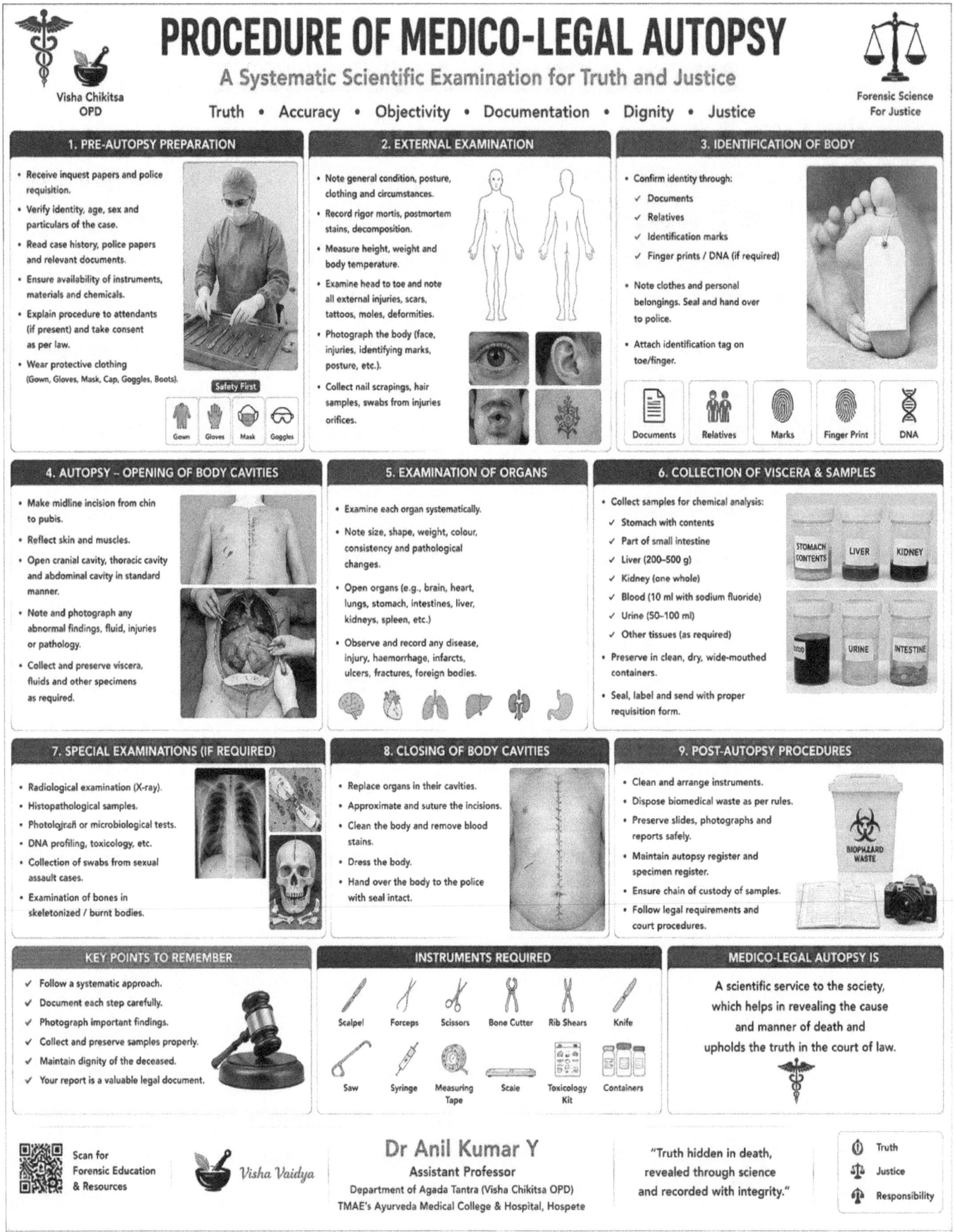
Visha Chikitsa OPD
PROCEDURE OF MEDICO-LEGAL AUTOPSY
A Systematic Scientific Examination for Truth and Justice
Truth • Accuracy • Objectivity • Documentation • Dignity • Justice
Forensic Science For Justice
1. PRE-AUTOPSY PREPARATION
• Receive inquest papers and police requisition.
• Verify identity, age, sex and particulars of the case.
• Read case history, police papers and relevant documents.
• Ensure availability of instruments, materials and chemicals.
• Explain procedure to attendants (if present) and take consent as per law.
• Wear protective clothing (Gown, Gloves, Mask, Cap, Goggles, Boots).
Safety First
Gown
Gloves
Mask
Goggles
2. EXTERNAL EXAMINATION
• Note general condition, posture, clothing and circumstances.
• Record rigor mortis, postmortem stains, decomposition.
• Measure height, weight and body temperature.
• Examine head to toe and note all external injuries, scars, tattoos, moles, deformities.
• Photograph the body (face, injuries, identifying marks, posture, etc.).
• Collect nail scrapings, hair samples, swabs from injuries orifices.
3. IDENTIFICATION OF BODY
• Confirm identity through:
✓ Documents
✓ Relatives
✓ Identification marks
✓ Finger prints / DNA (if required)
• Note clothes and personal belongings. Seal and hand over to police.
• Attach identification tag on toe/finger.
Documents
Relatives
Marks
Finger Print
DNA
4. AUTOPSY – OPENING OF BODY CAVITIES
• Make midline incision from chin to pubis.
• Reflect skin and muscles.
• Open cranial cavity, thoracic cavity and abdominal cavity in standard manner.
• Note and photograph any abnormal findings, fluid, injuries or pathology.
• Collect and preserve viscera, fluids and other specimens as required.
5. EXAMINATION OF ORGANS
• Examine each organ systematically.
• Note size, shape, weight, colour, consistency and pathological changes.
• Open organs (e.g., brain, heart, lungs, stomach, intestines, liver, kidneys, spleen, etc.)
• Observe and record any disease, injury, haemorrhage, infarcts, ulcers, fractures, foreign bodies.
6. COLLECTION OF VISCERA & SAMPLES
• Collect samples for chemical analysis:
✓ Stomach with contents
✓ Part of small intestine
✓ Liver (200–500 g)
✓ Kidney (one whole)
✓ Blood (10 ml with sodium fluoride)
✓ Urine (50–100 ml)
✓ Other tissues (as required)
• Preserve in clean, dry, wide-mouthed containers.
• Seal, label and send with proper requisition form.
STOMACH CONTENTS
LIVER
KIDNEY
URINE
INTESTINE
7. SPECIAL EXAMINATIONS (IF REQUIRED)
• Radiological examination (X-ray).
• Histopathological samples.
• Photolojrafi or microbiological tests.
• DNA profiling, toxicology, etc.
• Collection of swabs from sexual assault cases.
• Examination of bones in skeletonized / burnt bodies.
8. CLOSING OF BODY CAVITIES
• Replace organs in their cavities.
• Approximate and suture the incisions.
• Clean the body and remove blood stains.
• Dress the body.
• Hand over the body to the police with seal intact.
9. POST-AUTOPSY PROCEDURES
• Clean and arrange instruments.
• Dispose biomedical waste as per rules.
• Preserve slides, photographs and reports safely.
• Maintain autopsy register and specimen register.
• Ensure chain of custody of samples.
• Follow legal requirements and court procedures.
BIOHAZARD WASTE
KEY POINTS TO REMEMBER
✓ Follow a systematic approach.
✓ Document each step carefully.
✓ Photograph important findings.
✓ Collect and preserve samples properly.
✓ Maintain dignity of the deceased.
✓ Your report is a valuable legal document.
INSTRUMENTS REQUIRED
Scalpel
Forceps
Scissors
Bone Cutter
Rib Shears
Knife
Saw
Syringe
Measuring Tape
Scale
Toxicology Kit
Containers
MEDICO-LEGAL AUTOPSY IS
A scientific service to the society, which helps in revealing the cause and manner of death and upholds the truth in the court of law.
Scan for Forensic Education & Resources
Visha Vaidya
Dr Anil Kumar Y
Assistant Professor
Department of Agada Tantra (Visha Chikitsa OPD)
TMAE's Ayurveda Medical College & Hospital, Hospete
"Truth hidden in death, revealed through science and recorded with integrity."
Truth
Justice
Responsibility

PRACTICAL NO. 12

THANATOLOGY

OBSERVATION OF MEDICO-LEGAL AUTOPSY AND PREPARATION OF AUTOPSY REPORT

CASE 1:

Date: __________

Aim

To observe the procedure of medico-legal autopsy and understand the preparation of an autopsy report.

Objectives

1. To observe the external and internal examination of a dead body.
2. To understand the medico-legal importance of autopsy.
3. To learn the method of collection and preservation of viscera.
4. To study the preparation of an autopsy report.

Observations

Particulars of the Case

- PM No.: __________________
- Name of Deceased: __________________
- Age/Sex: __________________
- Date & Time of Autopsy: __________________
- Place of Autopsy: __________________
- Conducted By: __________________

Procedure Observed

1. Verification

- Identification of the body was confirmed.
- Police requisition and relevant documents were verified.

2. External Examination

- Age, sex and built of the deceased noted.
- Clothing examined and described.
- Identification marks recorded.
- Postmortem changes observed.

- External injuries noted and measured.

3. Internal Examination

- Scalp and skull examined.
- Thoracic cavity opened and organs examined.
- Abdominal cavity opened and organs examined.
- Cranial cavity opened and brain examined.

4. Preservation of Viscera

- Stomach and contents.
- Small intestine and contents.
- Liver and kidney samples.
- Blood and urine samples (if required).

5. Documentation

- Findings recorded systematically.
- Cause of death assessed.
- Opinion reserved if chemical analysis awaited.

Findings

Examination	Observation
External Appearance	____________________
Postmortem Changes	____________________
External Injuries	____________________
Internal Findings	____________________
Viscera Preserved	____________________
Probable Cause of Death	____________________

Sample Autopsy Opinion

"Based on the autopsy findings, death appears to be due to ___________________________. Final opinion is subject to chemical analysis report, if applicable."

Learning Points

1. Medico-legal autopsy helps ascertain the cause of death.
2. External and internal examinations are conducted systematically.
3. Proper preservation of viscera is essential in suspected poisoning cases.
4. Autopsy findings assist courts and investigating agencies.
5. Autopsy report is an important medico-legal document.

Result

Observed the medico-legal autopsy procedure and understood the preparation of an autopsy report including external examination, internal examination, viscera preservation and formulation of opinion regarding cause of death.

Teacher's Signature

Student's Signature

PRACTICAL NO. 12

THANATOLOGY

OBSERVATION OF MEDICO-LEGAL AUTOPSY AND PREPARATION OF AUTOPSY REPORT

CASE 2:

Date: __________

Aim

To observe the procedure of medico-legal autopsy and understand the preparation of an autopsy report.

Objectives

5. To observe the external and internal examination of a dead body.
6. To understand the medico-legal importance of autopsy.
7. To learn the method of collection and preservation of viscera.
8. To study the preparation of an autopsy report.

Observations

Particulars of the Case

- PM No.: __________________
- Name of Deceased: __________________
- Age/Sex: __________________
- Date & Time of Autopsy: __________________
- Place of Autopsy: __________________
- Conducted By: __________________

Procedure Observed

1. Verification

- Identification of the body was confirmed.
- Police requisition and relevant documents were verified.

2. External Examination

- Age, sex and built of the deceased noted.
- Clothing examined and described.
- Identification marks recorded.
- Postmortem changes observed.

- External injuries noted and measured.

3. Internal Examination

- Scalp and skull examined.
- Thoracic cavity opened and organs examined.
- Abdominal cavity opened and organs examined.
- Cranial cavity opened and brain examined.

4. Preservation of Viscera

- Stomach and contents.
- Small intestine and contents.
- Liver and kidney samples.
- Blood and urine samples (if required).

5. Documentation

- Findings recorded systematically.
- Cause of death assessed.
- Opinion reserved if chemical analysis awaited.

Findings

Examination	Observation
External Appearance	____________________
Postmortem Changes	____________________
External Injuries	____________________
Internal Findings	____________________
Viscera Preserved	____________________
Probable Cause of Death	____________________

Sample Autopsy Opinion

"Based on the autopsy findings, death appears to be due to ______________________. Final opinion is subject to chemical analysis report, if applicable."

Learning Points

6. Medico-legal autopsy helps ascertain the cause of death.
7. External and internal examinations are conducted systematically.
8. Proper preservation of viscera is essential in suspected poisoning cases.
9. Autopsy findings assist courts and investigating agencies.
10. Autopsy report is an important medico-legal document.

Result

Observed the medico-legal autopsy procedure and understood the preparation of an autopsy report including external examination, internal examination, viscera preservation and formulation of opinion regarding cause of death.

Teacher's Signature

Student's Signature

Visha Chikitsa OPD

DIFFERENCES BETWEEN HOMICIDAL, SUICIDAL & ACCIDENTAL INJURIES

Understanding the Nature of Injury – For Truth, Justice and Scientific Opinion

Forensic Science For Justice

BASIS FOR DIFFERENCE	HOMICIDAL INJURIES	SUICIDAL INJURIES	ACCIDENTAL INJURIES
INTENT	• Injury is inflicted by another person • with intention to cause harm or death.	• Injury is self-inflicted with intention • to cause harm or death.	• Injury occurs unintentionally, without any intention to cause harm or death.
NATURE OF INJURY	• Multiple injuries common • Defensive injuries usually present • Vital parts of body usually targeted (head, neck, chest, abdomen)	• Usually single or few injuries • Non-vital parts commonly chosen • Nature of injury depends on method used	• Variable • Depends on the nature of accident and instrument involved
SITE OF INJURY	• Injuries often on front of body • Vital organs commonly affected • Distribution varies	• Injuries often on accessible parts • Back of hands, wrists, side of neck, chest, abdomen etc.	• Injuries depend on mode of accident • Any part of body may be affected
DEFENSIVE INJURIES	• Present • Seen on hands, forearms, fingers while resisting	• Absent (except in some cases like self-defense in hanging)	• Absent
NUMBER OF INJURIES	• Usually multiple • Different ages (fresh & old)	• Usually single or few • Generally of same age	• Usually single • Unless multiple accidents occur
DIRECTION & NATURE	• Injuries from different directions • May show hesitation marks in sharp force injuries	• Injuries have definite direction • Hesitation marks may be present in cut throat	• Corresponds to the force and direction of the agent involved in accident
WEAPON / AGENT USED	• Any weapon • Choice depends on availability and knowledge	• Commonly available means used • Hanging, poisoning, self-cutting, firearm etc.	• Depends on the nature of accident • Road traffic accidents, falls, burns, drowning etc.
ASSOCIATED FINDINGS	• Signs of struggle • Disarranged clothes • Presence of other persons	• Suicide note may be present • Preparatory acts may be present • Solitary place	• No struggle • Scene suggests accident • No preparatory acts
SCENE OF OCCURRENCE	• Often away from place of occurrence • Signs of struggle, blood stains, drag marks etc.	• Usually at the place of occurrence • May be in secluded place	• Usually at the place of occurrence • Scene suggests accidental nature

EXAMPLES

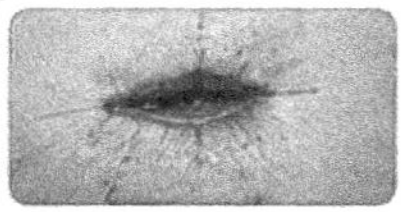
Multiple stab injuries on front of chest

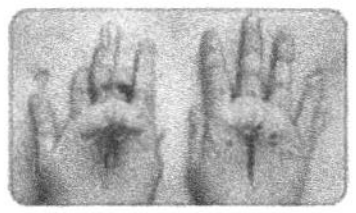
Defensive injuries on hands

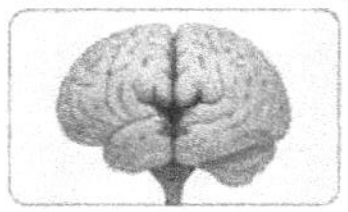
Injury to vital organs (Brain)

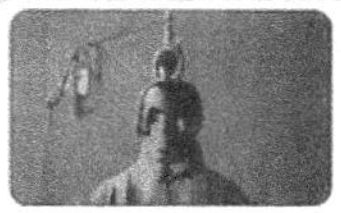
Hanging – ligature mark on neck

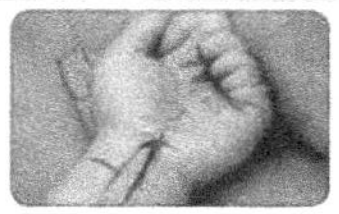
Cut injuries on wrist (self-inflicted)

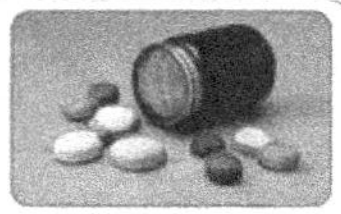
Poisoning – tablets and note

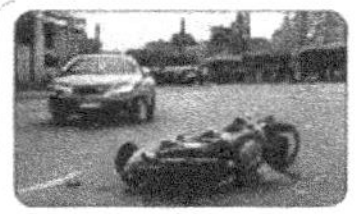
Road traffic accident

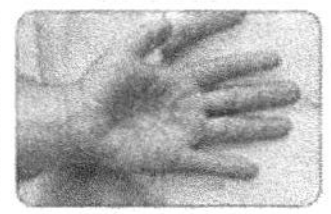
Burn injury due to fire

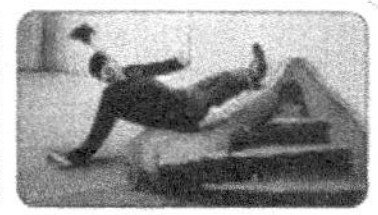
Fall from height / ground level

NOTE: Opinion should be based on careful consideration of all findings, circumstances and evidence.

"Truth is hidden in details, Science reveals the truth."

- Proper history
- Thorough examination
- Careful documentation
- Scientific approach
- Objectivity
- Justice

PRACTICAL NO. 13

DEMONSTRATION OF DIFFERENCE BETWEEN HOMICIDAL, SUICIDAL AND ACCIDENTAL INJURIES

Aim

To study and differentiate homicidal, suicidal and accidental injuries based on their characteristics and medico-legal findings.

Objectives

1. To identify the nature of injuries.
2. To understand the medico-legal significance of injury patterns.
3. To differentiate between homicidal, suicidal and accidental injuries.

Observations

Feature	Homicidal Injury	Suicidal Injury	Accidental Injury
Definition	Injury inflicted by another person with intent to harm	Self-inflicted injury with intent to end life	Injury occurring unintentionally
Number of Injuries	Usually multiple	Usually single or few	Variable
Site of Injury	Any accessible or inaccessible part	Accessible parts of body	Exposed parts of body
Hesitation Cuts	Absent	Present (especially in cut throat/wrist cases)	Absent
Defence Injuries	Commonly present	Absent	Usually absent
Clothing Damage	Often present	Usually absent or minimal	May be present
Direction of Injury	Variable	Follows natural hand movement	Variable
Weapon	Often removed or concealed	Usually found near victim	Depends on incident
Scene Findings	Signs of struggle may be present	Suicide note may be present	Evidence of accident present

Feature	Homicidal Injury	Suicidal Injury	Accidental Injury
Medico-Legal Nature	Crime against person	Self-inflicted act	Unintentional event

Key Identification Features

Homicidal Injuries

- Multiple injuries.
- Defence wounds on hands and forearms.
- Signs of struggle.
- Injuries may involve inaccessible parts of body.
- Weapon may be absent from scene.

Suicidal Injuries

- Hesitation cuts present.
- Injury on accessible body parts.
- Usually single fatal wound.
- Weapon often found nearby.
- No defence injuries.

Accidental Injuries

- Correspond to circumstances of accident.
- Irregular abrasions, contusions and lacerations common.
- No hesitation cuts.
- No defence wounds.
- Injuries often on exposed body parts.

Result

The differences between homicidal, suicidal and accidental injuries were observed and understood based on injury pattern, location, associated findings and medico-legal significance.

Conclusion

Careful examination of the type, number, location and characteristics of injuries helps in differentiating homicidal, suicidal and accidental injuries and assists in medico-legal investigation.

Teacher's Signature

Student's Signature

PRACTICAL NO. 13

DEMONSTRATION OF DIFFERENCE BETWEEN HOMICIDAL, SUICIDAL AND ACCIDENTAL INJURIES
DEMONSTRATION OF DRAFTING OF AN INJURY REPORT

Aim

To observe and learn the procedure for drafting a medico-legal injury report.

Objectives

1. To understand the components of an injury report.
2. To learn documentation of injuries in medico-legal cases.
3. To know the medico-legal importance of injury certification.

Observation

Particulars Recorded

- Name of Patient: ___________________
- Age/Sex: ___________________
- Address: ___________________
- MLC No.: ___________________
- Date and Time of Examination: ___________________
- Identification Marks: ___________________

General Examination

- Consciousness: Present / Absent
- Pulse: __________
- Blood Pressure: __________
- General Condition: Stable / Unstable

Injury Examination

Sl. No.	Nature of Injury	Site	Size	Remarks
1	Abrasion / Contusion / Laceration / Incised wound	__________	__________	__________
2	__________	__________	__________	__________

Opinion

- Nature of injury: Simple / Grievous
- Age of injury: __________
- Weapon used: Blunt / Sharp / Not known
- Dangerous to life: Yes / No

Sample Injury Report

INJURY CERTIFICATE

MLC No.: __________

Date & Time: __________

Name of Patient: __________________

Age/Sex: __________________

Address: __________________

Brought by: Police / Relative / Self

Injuries Noted

1. Abrasion measuring 3 cm × 1 cm over the right forearm, reddish in colour.
2. Contusion measuring 5 cm × 2 cm over the left shoulder, bluish-black in colour.

Opinion

1. The injuries are simple in nature.
2. The injuries appear to have been caused by a blunt object.
3. The age of injuries is approximately within 24 hours.

Signature of Medical Officer

(Name & Seal)

Learning Points

1. Every injury must be described accurately regarding site, size and nature.
2. Use objective findings and avoid assumptions.
3. Injury reports are important medico-legal documents.
4. Opinion should be based on examination findings.

Result

Observed the procedure of drafting an injury report and learned the documentation of injuries, assessment of their nature, probable weapon and medico-legal opinion.

Teacher's Signature

Student's Signature

PRACTICAL NO. 13

DEMONSTRATION OF DIFFERENCE BETWEEN HOMICIDAL, SUICIDAL AND ACCIDENTAL INJURIES

DEMONSTRATION OF DRAFTING OF AN INJURY REPORT

Aim

Objectives

Observation

Particulars Recorded

- Name of Patient: __________________
- Age/Sex: __________________
- Address: __________________
- MLC No.: __________________
- Date and Time of Examination: __________________
- Identification Marks: __________________

General Examination

- Consciousness: Present / Absent
- Pulse: __________
- Blood Pressure: __________
- General Condition: Stable / Unstable

Injury Examination

Sl. No.	Nature of Injury	Site	Size	Remarks
1	Abrasion / Contusion / Laceration / Incised wound	__________	__________	__________
2	__________	__________	__________	__________

Opinion

- Nature of injury: Simple / Grievous
- Age of injury: __________
- Weapon used: Blunt / Sharp / Not known
- Dangerous to life: Yes / No

Sample Injury Report

INJURY CERTIFICATE

MLC No.: __________

Date & Time: __________

Name of Patient: __________________

Age/Sex: __________________

Address: __________________

Brought by: Police / Relative / Self

Injuries Noted

Opinion

Signature of Medical Officer

(Name & Seal)

Result

Teacher's Signature

Student's Signature

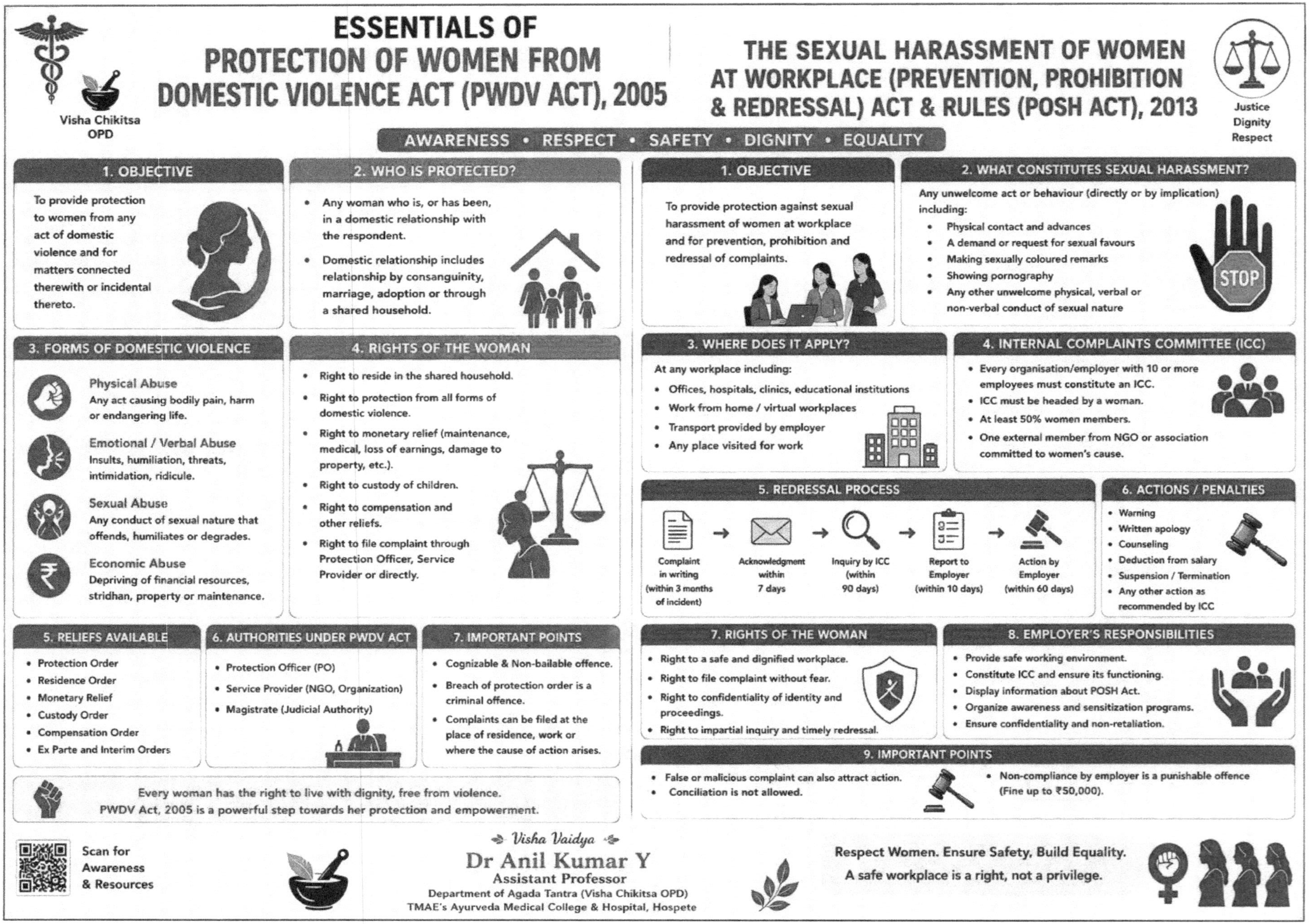
Visha Chikitsa OPD
ESSENTIALS OF
PROTECTION OF WOMEN FROM DOMESTIC VIOLENCE ACT (PWDV ACT), 2005
THE SEXUAL HARASSMENT OF WOMEN AT WORKPLACE (PREVENTION, PROHIBITION & REDRESSAL) ACT & RULES (POSH ACT), 2013
Justice Dignity Respect
AWARENESS • RESPECT • SAFETY • DIGNITY • EQUALITY
1. OBJECTIVE
To provide protection to women from any act of domestic violence and for matters connected therewith or incidental thereto.
2. WHO IS PROTECTED?
• Any woman who is, or has been, in a domestic relationship with the respondent.
• Domestic relationship includes relationship by consanguinity, marriage, adoption or through a shared household.
3. FORMS OF DOMESTIC VIOLENCE
Physical Abuse
Any act causing bodily pain, harm or endangering life.
Emotional / Verbal Abuse
Insults, humiliation, threats, intimidation, ridicule.
Sexual Abuse
Any conduct of sexual nature that offends, humiliates or degrades.
Economic Abuse
Depriving of financial resources, stridhan, property or maintenance.
4. RIGHTS OF THE WOMAN
• Right to reside in the shared household.
• Right to protection from all forms of domestic violence.
• Right to monetary relief (maintenance, medical, loss of earnings, damage to property, etc.).
• Right to custody of children.
• Right to compensation and other reliefs.
• Right to file complaint through Protection Officer, Service Provider or directly.
5. RELIEFS AVAILABLE
• Protection Order
• Residence Order
• Monetary Relief
• Custody Order
• Compensation Order
• Ex Parte and Interim Orders
6. AUTHORITIES UNDER PWDV ACT
• Protection Officer (PO)
• Service Provider (NGO, Organization)
• Magistrate (Judicial Authority)
7. IMPORTANT POINTS
• Cognizable & Non-bailable offence.
• Breach of protection order is a criminal offence.
• Complaints can be filed at the place of residence, work or where the cause of action arises.
Every woman has the right to live with dignity, free from violence.
PWDV Act, 2005 is a powerful step towards her protection and empowerment.
1. OBJECTIVE
To provide protection against sexual harassment of women at workplace and for prevention, prohibition and redressal of complaints.
2. WHAT CONSTITUTES SEXUAL HARASSMENT?
Any unwelcome act or behaviour (directly or by implication) including:
• Physical contact and advances
• A demand or request for sexual favours
• Making sexually coloured remarks
• Showing pornography
• Any other unwelcome physical, verbal or non-verbal conduct of sexual nature
STOP
3. WHERE DOES IT APPLY?
At any workplace including:
• Offices, hospitals, clinics, educational institutions
• Work from home / virtual workplaces
• Transport provided by employer
• Any place visited for work
4. INTERNAL COMPLAINTS COMMITTEE (ICC)
• Every organisation/employer with 10 or more employees must constitute an ICC.
• ICC must be headed by a woman.
• At least 50% women members.
• One external member from NGO or association committed to women's cause.
5. REDRESSAL PROCESS
Complaint in writing (within 3 months of incident)
Acknowledgment within 7 days
Inquiry by ICC (within 90 days)
Report to Employer (within 10 days)
Action by Employer (within 60 days)
6. ACTIONS / PENALTIES
• Warning
• Written apology
• Counseling
• Deduction from salary
• Suspension / Termination
• Any other action as recommended by ICC
7. RIGHTS OF THE WOMAN
• Right to a safe and dignified workplace.
• Right to file complaint without fear.
• Right to confidentiality of identity and proceedings.
• Right to impartial inquiry and timely redressal.
8. EMPLOYER'S RESPONSIBILITIES
• Provide safe working environment.
• Constitute ICC and ensure its functioning.
• Display information about POSH Act.
• Organize awareness and sensitization programs.
• Ensure confidentiality and non-retaliation.
9. IMPORTANT POINTS
• False or malicious complaint can also attract action.
• Conciliation is not allowed.
• Non-compliance by employer is a punishable offence (Fine up to ₹50,000).
Scan for Awareness & Resources
Visha Vaidya
Dr Anil Kumar Y
Assistant Professor
Department of Agada Tantra (Visha Chikitsa OPD)
TMAE's Ayurveda Medical College & Hospital, Hospete
Respect Women. Ensure Safety, Build Equality.
A safe workplace is a right, not a privilege.

PRACTICAL NO. 14

DISCUSSION ON THE ESSENTIALS OF THE PROTECTION OF WOMEN FROM DOMESTIC VIOLENCE (PWDV) ACT, 2005

Aim

To study and discuss the essential provisions of the Protection of Women from Domestic Violence (PWDV) Act, 2005.

Objectives

1. To understand the concept of domestic violence.
2. To know the rights and remedies available to women under the Act.
3. To understand the role of Protection Officers and Magistrates.
4. To study various orders granted under the Act.

Introduction

The Protection of Women from Domestic Violence Act, 2005 was enacted to provide effective protection to women who are subjected to violence within the family or domestic relationship. The Act recognizes physical, sexual, verbal, emotional and economic abuse as forms of domestic violence.

Essentials of the PWDV Act, 2005

Sl. No.	Provision	Observation
1	Aggrieved Person	Any woman who is or has been in a domestic relationship and alleges domestic violence.
2	Domestic Relationship	Relationship through marriage, blood, adoption, family relationship or relationship in the nature of marriage.
3	Domestic Violence	Includes physical, sexual, verbal, emotional and economic abuse.
4	Shared Household	Woman has the right to reside in the shared household.
5	Protection Officer	Assists the victim and coordinates with court, police and medical facilities.
6	Protection Order	Prevents further acts of violence by the respondent.
7	Residence Order	Protects the right of residence and may provide alternate accommodation.

Sl. No.	Provision	Observation
8	Monetary Relief	Compensation for expenses and losses suffered due to violence.
9	Custody Order	Temporary custody of children may be granted by the Magistrate.
10	Compensation Order	Compensation may be awarded for injuries and mental trauma.

Role of Medical Practitioner

- Examine and treat the victim.
- Document injuries accurately.
- Prepare Medico-Legal Case (MLC) records when required.
- Preserve evidence.
- Provide medical reports to investigating authorities.

Learning Points

1. Domestic violence includes more than physical assault.
2. The Act provides civil remedies and immediate protection.
3. Women have a right to reside in the shared household.
4. Protection Officers play an important role in implementation.
5. Medical documentation is important for legal proceedings.

Result

The essential provisions of the Protection of Women from Domestic Violence Act, 2005 were studied and understood, including the rights of aggrieved women, types of relief available and the medico-legal role of healthcare professionals.

Conclusion

The PWDV Act, 2005 is an important social welfare legislation that provides legal protection, residence rights, monetary relief and other remedies to women affected by domestic violence, ensuring their safety and dignity.

Teacher's Signature

Student's Signature

PRACTICAL NO. 14

DISCUSSION ON THE SEXUAL HARASSMENT OF WOMEN AT WORKPLACE (PREVENTION, PROHIBITION AND REDRESSAL) ACT, 2013

Aim

To study and discuss the provisions of the Sexual Harassment of Women at Workplace (Prevention, Prohibition and Redressal) Act, 2013.

Objectives

1. To understand the concept of sexual harassment at the workplace.
2. To know the preventive and redressal mechanisms under the Act.
3. To understand the constitution and functions of the Internal Committee.
4. To recognize the role of employers in ensuring a safe workplace.

Introduction

The Sexual Harassment of Women at Workplace (Prevention, Prohibition and Redressal) Act, 2013 (POSH Act) was enacted to provide protection against sexual harassment of women at workplaces and to ensure a safe, secure and dignified working environment.

Essentials of the Act

Sl. No.	Provision	Observation
1	Objective	Protection of women from sexual harassment at workplace
2	Aggrieved Woman	Any woman alleging sexual harassment at workplace
3	Workplace	Includes hospitals, educational institutions, offices, clinics and other workplaces
4	Sexual Harassment	Unwelcome physical, verbal or non-verbal conduct of a sexual nature
5	Internal Committee (IC)	Mandatory in establishments with 10 or more employees
6	Local Committee (LC)	Constituted at district level where IC is not available

Sl. No.	Provision	Observation
7	Complaint	Written complaint to be made within prescribed time
8	Inquiry Process	Conducted by Internal Committee or Local Committee
9	Interim Relief	Transfer, leave or other relief during inquiry
10	Action on Complaint	Disciplinary action if allegations are proved

What Constitutes Sexual Harassment?

- Unwelcome physical contact and advances.
- Demand or request for sexual favours.
- Sexually coloured remarks.
- Showing pornography.
- Any unwelcome physical, verbal or non-verbal conduct of a sexual nature.

Internal Committee (IC)

Composition

- Presiding Officer – Senior woman employee.
- At least two employee members.
- One external member familiar with women's issues or legal matters.

Functions

- Receive complaints.
- Conduct inquiry.
- Recommend action.
- Maintain confidentiality.

Duties of Employer

1. Provide a safe working environment.
2. Display provisions of the Act prominently.
3. Organize awareness programmes.
4. Assist the Internal Committee.
5. Take appropriate action on recommendations.

Role of Medical Professionals

- Maintain professional conduct.
- Ensure respectful workplace behaviour.
- Report incidents through proper channels.
- Cooperate with inquiry proceedings when required.
- Promote awareness regarding workplace safety.

Learning Points

1. Sexual harassment is a violation of dignity and fundamental rights.
2. Every workplace should have a mechanism for redressal.
3. Hospitals and medical colleges are covered under the Act.
4. Confidentiality of complaints must be maintained.
5. Awareness and prevention are essential for a safe workplace.

Result

The provisions of the Sexual Harassment of Women at Workplace (Prevention, Prohibition and Redressal) Act, 2013 were studied and understood, including complaint procedures, preventive measures, and redressal mechanisms.

Conclusion

The Act aims to ensure a safe, secure and dignified work environment for women by preventing sexual harassment, providing a mechanism for complaint redressal and promoting gender equality at the workplace.

Teacher's Signature

Student's Signature

FORENSIC SCIENCE LABORATORY (FSL)

APPRISE THE FUNCTIONING OF A FORENSIC SCIENCE LABORATORY

Visha Chikitsa OPD

Forensic Science For Justice

"SCIENCE SERVES JUSTICE – TRUTH, EVIDENCE, INTEGRITY"

1. INTRODUCTION

The Forensic Science Laboratory is a specialized institution that applies scientific methods and technology to examine and analyze evidence collected from crime scenes. It provides objective, reliable and admissible results to assist the investigation agencies and the court of law.

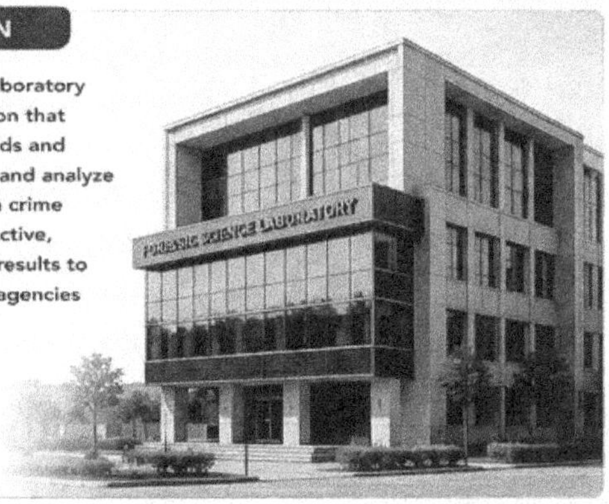

2. OBJECTIVES

- To collect, preserve and analyze physical evidence.
- To provide scientific and objective opinion.
- To aid in the investigation and detection of crime.
- To present findings in court.
- To uphold justice through science.

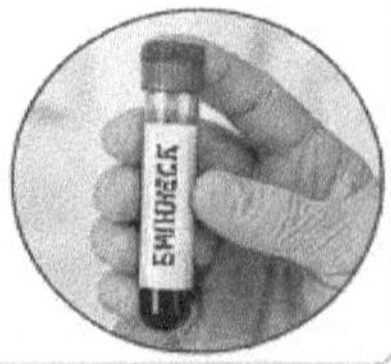

3. STRUCTURE OF FSL

- Director / Head (Overall Incharge)
- Scientific Officers & Experts
- Technical Staff
- Administrative Staff
- Support Staff

4. MAJOR DIVISIONS / SECTIONS IN FSL

PHYSICAL SCIENCE SECTION
- Document examination
- Questioned handwriting
- Fingerprints
- Tool mark analysis
- Age determination
- Ballistics

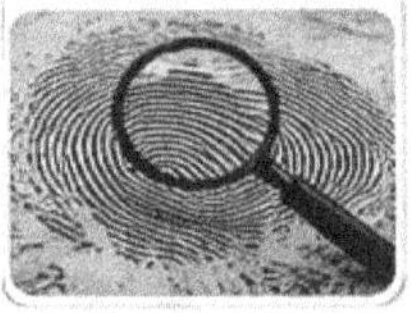

CHEMICAL SECTION
- Poison analysis
- Narcotic drugs
- Toxicology
- Explosives
- Arson residues
- Trace evidence

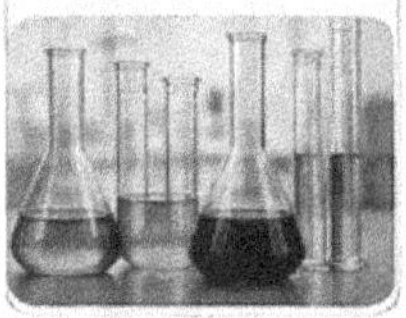

BIOLOGICAL SECTION
- Blood, semen, saliva analysis
- DNA profiling
- Hair analysis
- Serology

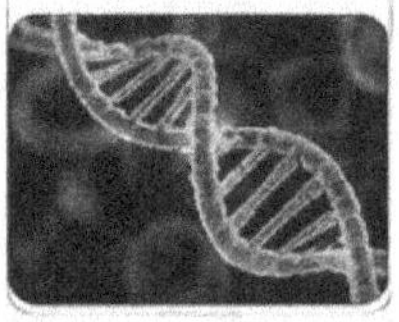

DOCUMENT & QUESTIONED ITEM SECTION
- Forged documents
- Ink & paper examination
- Stamp & seal analysis
- Currency verification

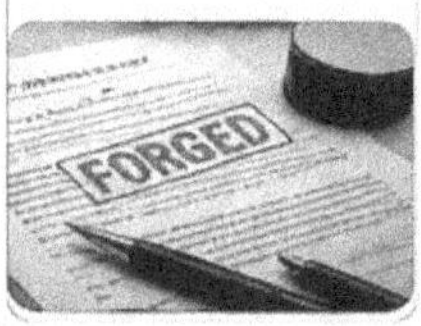

BALLISTICS SECTION
- Firearms
- Ammunition
- Bullet recovery
- Trajectory analysis

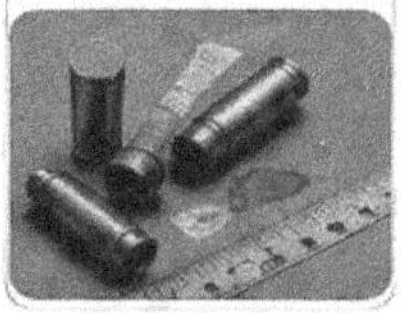

DIGITAL FORENSICS SECTION
- Mobile & computer forensics
- Data recovery
- Cyber crime evidence
- Multimedia analysis

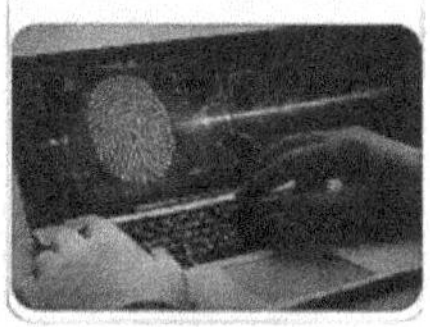

5. FUNCTIONING / WORK FLOW

RECEIPT OF EXHIBITS → REGISTRATION → EXAMINATION & ANALYSIS → DOCUMENTATION → REPORT PREPARATION → DISPATCH & COURT TESTIMONY

RECEIPT OF EXHIBITS	Sealed exhibits received from investigating officers with proper form & acknowledgement
REGISTRATION	Unique case number is allotted. Details entered in exhibit register and case file opened.
EXAMINATION & ANALYSIS	Scientific examination using standard methods and instruments in respective sections.
DOCUMENTATION	Observations, tests, results and opinions are recorded in case notes and work sheets.
REPORT PREPARATION	Expert opinion is compiled, reviewed and signed by the competent authority.
DISPATCH & COURT TESTIMONY	Report sent to investigating authority. Expert may be called to court as witness.

6. QUALITY & STANDARD PRACTICES

- ✓ Follows Standard Operating Procedures (SOPs).
- ✓ Use of validated scientific methods and calibrated instruments.
- ✓ Chain of custody maintained.
- ✓ Internal quality control & proficiency testing.
- ✓ Confidentiality, Impartiality & Integrity ensured.
- ✓ Accreditation as per ISO/IEC 17025.

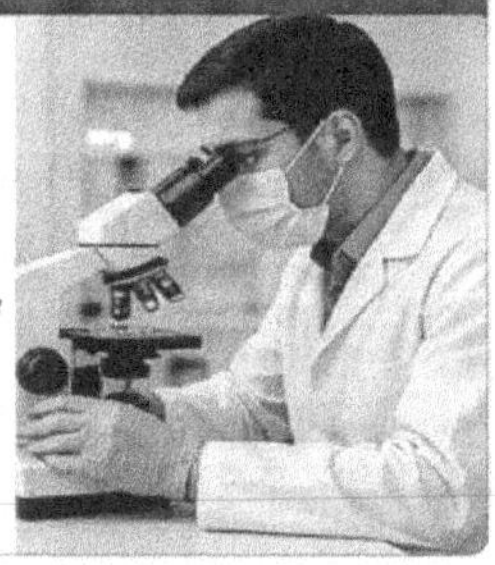

7. IMPORTANCE OF FSL

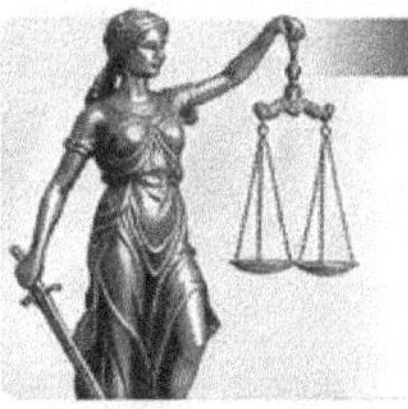

- ✓ Provides scientific and objective evidence.
- ✓ Helps in solving crimes and identifying offenders.
- ✓ Supports fair investigation and prosecution.
- ✓ Prevents miscarriage of justice.
- ✓ Strengthens the rule of law and public trust.

8. MODERN TECHNOLOGIES IN FSL

- DNA Profiling
- LC-MS / GC-MS Analysis
- AFIS (Fingerprint Identification)
- Digital & Cyber Forensics Tools
- 3D Scanning & Imaging
- Spectroscopy & Microscopy

9. ETHICS IN FORENSIC SCIENCE

- **INTEGRITY** – Maintain honesty and truthfulness in all findings.
- **IMPARTIALITY** – No bias or influence in analysis and opinion.
- **CONFIDENTIALITY** – Maintain secrecy of case details and reports.
- **COMPETENCE** – Work within the limits of expertise and training.
- **ACCOUNTABILITY** – Accept reponsibility for the results and opinions given.
- **RESPECT FOR LAW** – Support the legal process and human rights.

Scan for Forensic Education & Resources

Visha Vaidya

Dr Anil Kumar Y
Assistant Professor
Department of Agada Tantra (Visha Chikitsa OPD)
TMAE's Ayurveda Medical College & Hospital, Hospete

"When science speaks, Justice listens."

PRACTICAL NO. 15

FIELD VISIT REPORT

APPRAISAL OF THE FUNCTIONING OF A FORENSIC SCIENCE LABORATORY (FSL)

(Mandatory Practical Activity)

Date of Visit: __________

Place of Visit: ______________________

Name of Forensic Science Laboratory: ______________________

Accompanied By: ______________________

1. Title of Visit

Visit to Forensic Science Laboratory (FSL) for Appraisal of its Functioning.

2. Objectives

1. To understand the organization and functioning of a Forensic Science Laboratory.
2. To observe various forensic divisions and their roles.
3. To understand the scientific examination of medico-legal evidence.
4. To study the importance of forensic investigations in the administration of justice.

3. Introduction

A Forensic Science Laboratory (FSL) is a scientific institution that assists investigating agencies and courts by examining physical evidence collected from crime scenes. It applies scientific principles for the detection, analysis and interpretation of evidence.

4. Observations

A. General Information

- Name of Laboratory: ____________________
- Location: ____________________
- Date of Establishment: ____________________
- Authority Controlling the Laboratory: ____________________

B. Divisions/Sections Observed

Sl. No.	Division	Function
1	Biology/Serology Division	Examination of blood, semen, hair and biological samples
2	DNA Division	DNA profiling and identification
3	Toxicology Division	Analysis of poisons, drugs and toxic substances
4	Chemistry Division	Chemical analysis of evidence
5	Ballistics Division	Examination of firearms and ammunition
6	Fingerprint Division	Identification through fingerprints
7	Questioned Documents Division	Examination of handwriting, signatures and documents
8	Cyber Forensics Division	Analysis of digital evidence
9	Photography Division	Crime scene and evidence documentation

C. Evidence Examined

The following types of evidence were observed:

- Blood samples
- Hair samples
- Viscera samples
- Firearms and bullets
- Fingerprints
- Documents and signatures
- Digital devices
- Biological specimens

D. Procedure Observed

1. Receipt of evidence from investigating agencies.
2. Registration and labeling of exhibits.
3. Preservation and storage of samples.
4. Scientific examination and analysis.
5. Preparation of expert opinion.
6. Submission of forensic report to the concerned authority.

5. Importance of FSL

- Assists criminal investigation.
- Helps establish identity of victims and accused.
- Detects poisons and toxic substances.
- Provides scientific evidence in courts.
- Supports medico-legal investigations.

6. Learning Outcomes

1. Understood the organizational structure of FSL.
2. Observed different forensic divisions and their functions.
3. Learned the importance of scientific evidence in legal proceedings.
4. Understood the role of forensic experts in crime investigation.
5. Appreciated the significance of forensic science in medico-legal practice.

7. Conclusion

The visit to the Forensic Science Laboratory provided practical exposure to the scientific examination of evidence and the functioning of various forensic divisions. The visit enhanced understanding of the role of forensic science in criminal investigation, medico-legal cases and administration of justice.

8. Result

The functioning of the Forensic Science Laboratory was observed and understood, including evidence handling, analysis, reporting and its role in medico-legal and criminal investigations.

Teacher's Signature

Student's Signature

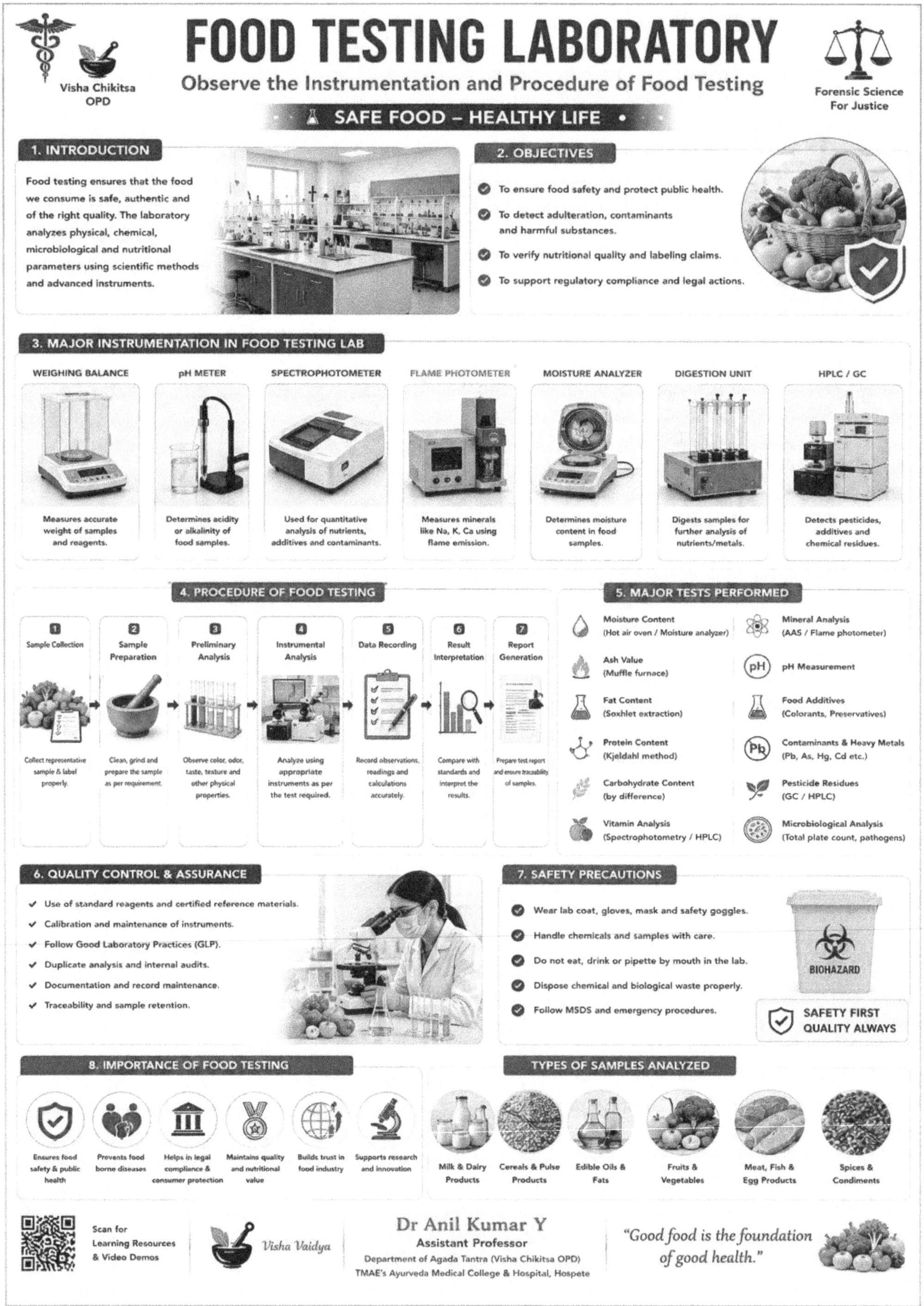
Visha Chikitsa OPD
FOOD TESTING LABORATORY
Observe the Instrumentation and Procedure of Food Testing
Forensic Science For Justice
SAFE FOOD – HEALTHY LIFE
1. INTRODUCTION
Food testing ensures that the food we consume is safe, authentic and of the right quality. The laboratory analyzes physical, chemical, microbiological and nutritional parameters using scientific methods and advanced instruments.
2. OBJECTIVES
To ensure food safety and protect public health.
To detect adulteration, contaminants and harmful substances.
To verify nutritional quality and labeling claims.
To support regulatory compliance and legal actions.
3. MAJOR INSTRUMENTATION IN FOOD TESTING LAB
WEIGHING BALANCE
Measures accurate weight of samples and reagents.
pH METER
Determines acidity or alkalinity of food samples.
SPECTROPHOTOMETER
Used for quantitative analysis of nutrients, additives and contaminants.
FLAME PHOTOMETER
Measures minerals like Na, K, Ca using flame emission.
MOISTURE ANALYZER
Determines moisture content in food samples.
DIGESTION UNIT
Digests samples for further analysis of nutrients/metals.
HPLC / GC
Detects pesticides, additives and chemical residues.
4. PROCEDURE OF FOOD TESTING
1 Sample Collection
Collect representative sample & label properly.
2 Sample Preparation
Clean, grind and prepare the sample as per requirement.
3 Preliminary Analysis
Observe color, odor, taste, texture and other physical properties.
4 Instrumental Analysis
Analyze using appropriate instruments as per the test required.
5 Data Recording
Record observations, readings and calculations accurately.
6 Result Interpretation
Compare with standards and interpret the results.
7 Report Generation
Prepare test report and ensure traceability of samples.
5. MAJOR TESTS PERFORMED
Moisture Content (Hot air oven / Moisture analyzer)
Mineral Analysis (AAS / Flame photometer)
Ash Value (Muffle furnace)
pH Measurement
Fat Content (Soxhlet extraction)
Food Additives (Colorants, Preservatives)
Protein Content (Kjeldahl method)
Contaminants & Heavy Metals (Pb, As, Hg, Cd etc.)
Carbohydrate Content (by difference)
Pesticide Residues (GC / HPLC)
Vitamin Analysis (Spectrophotometry / HPLC)
Microbiological Analysis (Total plate count, pathogens)
6. QUALITY CONTROL & ASSURANCE
Use of standard reagents and certified reference materials.
Calibration and maintenance of instruments.
Follow Good Laboratory Practices (GLP).
Duplicate analysis and internal audits.
Documentation and record maintenance.
Traceability and sample retention.
7. SAFETY PRECAUTIONS
Wear lab coat, gloves, mask and safety goggles.
Handle chemicals and samples with care.
Do not eat, drink or pipette by mouth in the lab.
Dispose chemical and biological waste properly.
Follow MSDS and emergency procedures.
BIOHAZARD
SAFETY FIRST QUALITY ALWAYS
8. IMPORTANCE OF FOOD TESTING
Ensures food safety & public health
Prevents food borne diseases
Helps in legal compliance & consumer protection
Maintains quality and nutritional value
Builds trust in food industry
Supports research and innovation
TYPES OF SAMPLES ANALYZED
Milk & Dairy Products
Cereals & Pulse Products
Edible Oils & Fats
Fruits & Vegetables
Meat, Fish & Egg Products
Spices & Condiments
Scan for Learning Resources & Video Demos
Visha Vaidya
Dr Anil Kumar Y
Assistant Professor
Department of Agada Tantra (Visha Chikitsa OPD)
TMAE's Ayurveda Medical College & Hospital, Hospete
"Good food is the foundation of good health."

PRACTICAL NO. 15

FIELD VISIT REPORT

VISIT TO FOOD TESTING LABORATORY – OBSERVATION OF INSTRUMENTATION AND PROCEDURE OF FOOD TESTING

Date of Visit: ___________

Place of Visit: ________________________

Name of Food Testing Laboratory: ________________________

Faculty Accompanying: ________________________

1. Title of Visit

Visit to Food Testing Laboratory to Observe the Instrumentation and Procedure of Food Testing.

2. Objectives

1. To understand the functioning of a food testing laboratory.
2. To observe instruments used for food analysis.
3. To study procedures adopted for testing food quality and safety.
4. To understand the role of food testing in public health.

3. Introduction

Food testing laboratories analyze food samples to determine their quality, purity, nutritional value and safety. These laboratories help detect adulterants, contaminants, toxins, microorganisms and chemical residues to ensure consumer safety.

4. Observations

A. General Information

- Name of Laboratory: ____________________
- Location: ____________________

- Accrediting Authority: ____________________
- Type of Laboratory: Government / Private

B. Instruments Observed

Sl. No.	Instrument	Purpose
1	pH Meter	Measurement of acidity/alkalinity
2	Analytical Balance	Accurate weighing of samples
3	UV-Visible Spectrophotometer	Chemical analysis of food constituents
4	High Performance Liquid Chromatography (HPLC)	Detection of additives, toxins and residues
5	Gas Chromatography (GC)	Analysis of pesticides and contaminants
6	Centrifuge	Separation of sample components
7	Hot Air Oven	Moisture determination
8	Incubator	Microbial culture growth
9	Microscope	Detection of adulterants and microorganisms
10	Autoclave	Sterilization of laboratory materials

C. Procedure Observed

1. Sample Collection

- Food samples received and registered.
- Unique identification number assigned.

2. Sample Preparation

- Homogenization and processing of food samples.
- Proper labeling and preservation.

3. Physical Examination

- Colour

- Odour
- Taste (where applicable)
- Texture and appearance

4. Chemical Analysis

- Moisture content
- Fat content
- Protein content
- Carbohydrate estimation
- Detection of preservatives and adulterants

5. Microbiological Testing

- Detection of bacterial contamination.
- Fungal and yeast examination.

6. Reporting

- Recording of observations.
- Comparison with food safety standards.
- Preparation of final laboratory report.

5. Common Food Adulterants Observed

Food Item	Possible Adulterant
Milk	Water, starch, detergent
Turmeric Powder	Metanil yellow
Chilli Powder	Brick powder, artificial colour
Tea Powder	Iron filings, used tea leaves
Ghee	Vanaspati
Honey	Sugar syrup

6. Learning Outcomes

1. Understood the workflow of a food testing laboratory.
2. Observed modern analytical instruments used in food analysis.

3. Learned procedures for detection of food adulteration.
4. Understood microbiological and chemical testing methods.
5. Appreciated the importance of food safety monitoring.

7. Conclusion

The visit provided practical exposure to food quality assessment, detection of adulteration and laboratory procedures used to ensure food safety. Food testing laboratories play a vital role in protecting public health and preventing food-borne hazards.

8. Result

Observed the instrumentation and procedures employed in a food testing laboratory, including sample collection, physical examination, chemical analysis, microbiological testing and preparation of food analysis reports.

Teacher's Signature

Student's Signature

Visha Chikitsa OPD

VISIT TO POLLUTION CONTROL BOARD

PERCEIVE THE FUNCTIONING OF POLLUTION CONTROL BOARD

Forensic Science For Justice

• • • CLEAN ENVIRONMENT – HEALTHY LIFE – SUSTAINABLE FUTURE • • •

1. INTRODUCTION

Pollution Control Board (PCB) is a statutory organization established under the Water (Prevention and Control of Pollution) Act, 1974 and Air (Prevention and Control of Pollution) Act, 1981.

It works to protect, improve and restore the environment by preventing and controlling pollution and ensuring sustainable development.

2. OBJECTIVES OF POLLUTION CONTROL BOARD

- To prevent, control and abate pollution of water, air and land.
- To promote cleanliness of streams and wells.
- To plan and execute nation-wide programmes for the prevention and control of pollution.
- To lay down standards for emission and discharge of pollutants.
- To grant consents and authorizations to industries.
- To spread awareness and promote environmental education.
- To collect, compile and publish environmental data.

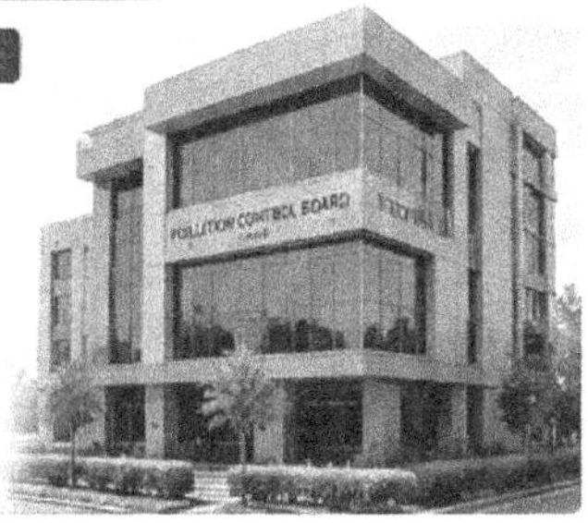

3. MAJOR FUNCTIONS / ACTIVITIES

STANDARDS SETTING	CONSENT MANAGEMENT	MONITORING & INSPECTION	SAMPLE COLLECTION & ANALYSIS	ENFORCEMENT OF LAW	RESEARCH & DEVELOPMENT	AWARENESS & TRAINING
Fixes standards for emissions, discharges and ambient quality.	Grants Consent to Establish (CTE) and Consent to Operate (CTO) to industries.	Regular inspection of industries and monitoring of pollution levels.	Collection of samples (water, air, soil, waste) and analysis in laboratories.	Taking legal action against defaulters under environmental laws.	Conducts research and develops new techniques for pollution control.	Spreads awareness and provides training for industries and public.

4. DEPARTMENTS / DIVISIONS IN PCB

- Administration
- Technical Division (Air)
- Technical Division (Water)
- Laboratory Division
- Legal Cell
- Monitoring Cell
- Environmental Engineering Division
- Public Relations & Awareness Cell

5. OBSERVATIONS DURING VISIT

- Understood the organizational structure and hierarchy.
- Observed the process of consent issuance.
- Visited laboratories and observed instruments used for sample analysis.
- Observed sampling procedure (air, water, soil, noise).
- Understood monitoring techniques and data recording.
- Interacted with technical experts and learned about environmental regulations.
- Realized the importance of environmental compliance by industries.

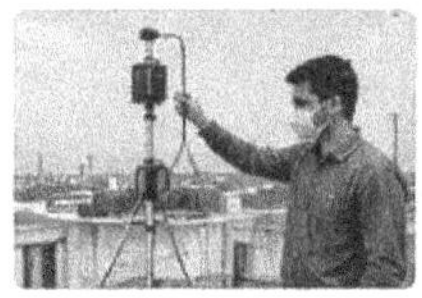

Air Sampling

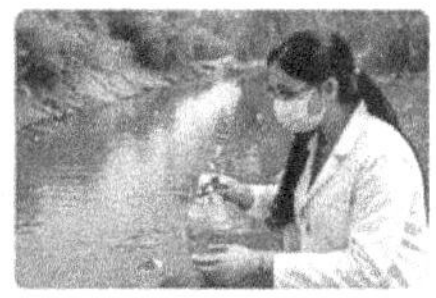

Water Sampling

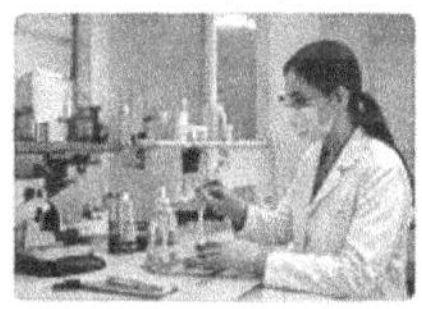

Laboratory Analysis

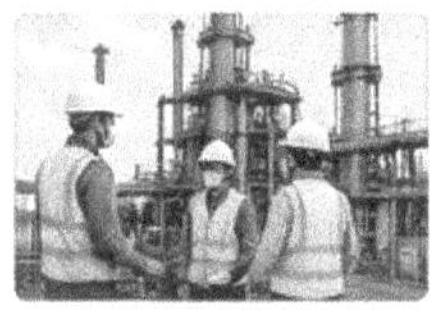

Industrial Inspection

6. LABORATORY INSTRUMENTS OBSERVED

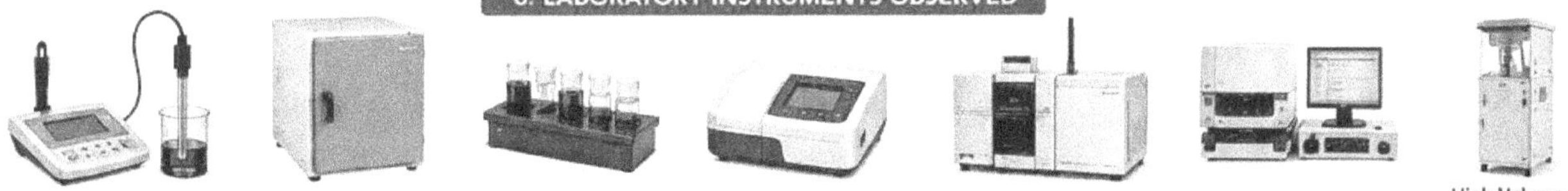

pH Meter | BOD Incubator | COD Reactor | Spectrophotometer | Gas Chromatograph | AAS / ICP-OES | High Volume Sampler

7. SAMPLING PROCEDURE (GENERAL STEPS)

Planning & Preparation → Collection of Sample → Preservation & Labeling → Transport to Laboratory → Analysis & Reporting

8. APPLICABLE LAWS & RULES

- Water (Prevention and Control of Pollution) Act, 1974
- Air (Prevention and Control of Pollution) Act, 1981
- Environment (Protection) Act, 1986
- Hazardous and Other Wastes (Management & Transboundary Movement) Rules, 2016
- E-Waste (Management) Rules, 2016
- Plastic Waste Management Rules, 2016

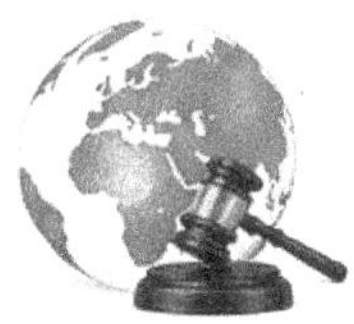

9. IMPORTANCE OF POLLUTION CONTROL BOARD

- Protects environment and public health.
- Ensures sustainable industrial development.
- Helps in climate change mitigation.
- Supports enforcement of environmental laws.
- Promotes clean air, clean water and green future.

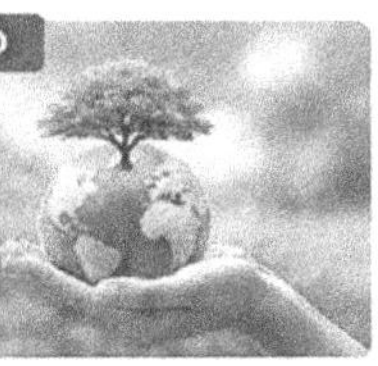

10. LEARNING OUTCOME

- Gained practical knowledge about the functioning of PCB.
- Understood the real-time process of environmental monitoring and analysis.
- Appreciated the role of PCB in maintaining ecological balance.
- Motivated to contribute towards a cleaner and greener society.

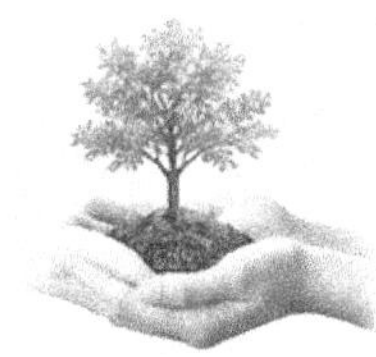

Scan for Environmental Education Resources

Visha Vaidya

Dr Anil Kumar Y
Assistant Professor
Department of Agada Tantra (Visha Chikitsa OPD)
TMAE's Ayurveda Medical College & Hospital, Hospete

"The Earth does not belong to us, we belong to the Earth."

Reduce
Reuse
Recycle
Respect

PRACTICAL NO. 15

FIELD VISIT REPORT

VISIT TO POLLUTION CONTROL BOARD (PCB)

(Mandatory Practical Activity)

Date of Visit: __________

Place of Visit: ______________________

Name of Pollution Control Board Office: ______________________

Faculty Accompanying: ______________________

1. Title of Visit

Visit to Pollution Control Board to Perceive its Functioning and Environmental Monitoring Activities.

2. Objectives

1. To understand the functioning of the Pollution Control Board.
2. To study environmental pollution monitoring activities.
3. To observe pollution control measures adopted for air, water and soil.
4. To understand the role of the Pollution Control Board in public health protection.

3. Introduction

The Pollution Control Board is a statutory organization responsible for prevention, control and monitoring of environmental pollution. It works towards maintaining environmental quality and safeguarding public health through enforcement of environmental laws and standards.

4. Observations

A. General Information

- Name of Office: ____________________
- Location: ____________________

- Type: Central Pollution Control Board (CPCB) / State Pollution Control Board (SPCB)
- Date of Visit: ____________________

B. Functions Observed

Sl. No.	Function	Observation
1	Air Pollution Control	Monitoring of ambient air quality
2	Water Pollution Control	Testing of water quality and effluents
3	Noise Pollution Monitoring	Measurement of environmental noise levels
4	Industrial Inspection	Inspection of industries for pollution compliance
5	Waste Management	Monitoring disposal of hazardous and biomedical waste
6	Environmental Awareness	Conducting educational and awareness programmes
7	Laboratory Analysis	Examination of environmental samples
8	Regulatory Activities	Granting consent and enforcing environmental laws

C. Laboratory/Monitoring Instruments Observed

Sl. No.	Instrument	Purpose
1	Air Quality Monitoring System	Monitoring air pollutants
2	pH Meter	Water quality analysis
3	Dissolved Oxygen (DO) Meter	Water pollution assessment
4	Sound Level Meter	Noise pollution monitoring
5	Spectrophotometer	Chemical analysis of samples
6	Gas Analyzer	Measurement of gaseous pollutants
7	Water Sampling Equipment	Collection of water samples
8	Particulate Matter Monitor	Monitoring $PM_{2.5}$ and PM_{10} levels

D. Environmental Samples Examined

- Air samples
- Water samples
- Industrial effluent samples
- Soil samples
- Noise level records

E. Procedure Observed

1. Collection of environmental samples.
2. Transportation and labeling of samples.
3. Laboratory analysis of pollutants.
4. Comparison with prescribed standards.
5. Preparation of analytical reports.
6. Regulatory action against violations.

5. Importance of Pollution Control Board

- Prevents environmental pollution.
- Protects public health.
- Monitors industrial emissions and effluents.
- Ensures compliance with environmental laws.
- Promotes sustainable development.

6. Learning Outcomes

1. Understood the structure and functioning of the Pollution Control Board.
2. Observed environmental monitoring activities.
3. Learned about laboratory testing of environmental samples.
4. Understood the role of pollution control in disease prevention.
5. Appreciated the importance of environmental protection for public health.

7. Conclusion

The visit provided practical exposure to environmental monitoring, pollution assessment and regulatory activities undertaken by the Pollution Control Board. The Board plays a vital role in controlling pollution and protecting environmental and public health.

8. Result

Observed and understood the functioning of the Pollution Control Board, including environmental monitoring, sample analysis, pollution control measures and enforcement of environmental regulations.

Teacher's Signature

Student's Signature

PRACTICAL NO. 15

FIELD VISIT REPORT

VISIT TO DE-ADDICTION CENTRE – OBSERVATION OF MANAGEMENT OF DE-ADDICTION CASES

Date of Visit: __________

Place of Visit: ______________________

Name of De-addiction Centre: ______________________

Faculty Accompanying: ______________________

1. Title of Visit

Visit to De-addiction Centre for Observation of Management of De-addiction Cases.

2. Objectives

1. To understand the functioning of a de-addiction centre.
2. To observe the assessment and management of substance dependence cases.
3. To study counselling and rehabilitation services.
4. To understand the role of healthcare professionals in addiction management.

3. Introduction

A De-addiction Centre provides treatment, counselling and rehabilitation services for individuals suffering from substance dependence such as alcohol, tobacco, opioids and other drugs. The centre aims to help patients achieve abstinence, improve health and reintegrate into society.

4. Observations

A. General Information

- Name of Centre: __________________
- Location: __________________

- Type of Centre: Government / Private
- Number of Beds: ____________________

B. Common Addiction Cases Observed

Sl. No.	Substance Dependence	Common Features
1	Alcohol Dependence	Tremors, craving, withdrawal symptoms
2	Tobacco Dependence	Nicotine craving, irritability
3	Opioid Dependence	Withdrawal symptoms, drug-seeking behaviour
4	Cannabis Dependence	Behavioural and psychological changes
5	Multiple Substance Abuse	Dependence on more than one substance

C. Management Procedure Observed

1. Registration and Assessment

- Patient registration.
- Detailed history taking.
- Physical and mental status examination.
- Assessment of substance use pattern.

2. Diagnosis

- Identification of substance dependence.
- Evaluation of severity of addiction.
- Screening for associated medical and psychiatric conditions.

3. Detoxification

- Management of withdrawal symptoms.
- Monitoring of vital signs.
- Supportive medical care.

4. Counselling Services

- Individual counselling.
- Family counselling.
- Motivational enhancement therapy.
- Relapse prevention counselling.

5. Rehabilitation

- Behavioural therapy.
- Group therapy sessions.
- Occupational and recreational activities.
- Social reintegration programmes.

6. Follow-Up

- Regular review visits.
- Monitoring for relapse.
- Continued psychological support.

5. Healthcare Team Observed

Professional	Role
Psychiatrist	Diagnosis and treatment
Medical Officer	Clinical management
Psychologist	Counselling and behavioural therapy
Social Worker	Family and social rehabilitation
Nursing Staff	Patient care and monitoring

6. Learning Outcomes

1. Understood the functioning of a de-addiction centre.
2. Observed assessment and treatment of addiction cases.
3. Learned the importance of counselling and rehabilitation.
4. Understood the multidisciplinary approach to addiction management.
5. Appreciated the importance of relapse prevention and follow-up care.

7. Conclusion

The visit provided practical exposure to the comprehensive management of substance dependence, including assessment, detoxification, counselling, rehabilitation and follow-up. Effective de-addiction management requires medical, psychological and social support.

8. Result

Observed the management of de-addiction cases, including patient assessment, detoxification, counselling, rehabilitation and follow-up services provided at the de-addiction centre.

Teacher's Signature

Student's Signature

Visha Chikitsa OPD

OBSERVE THE PROCEDURE OF COURT

PROCEDURE AND CONDUCT OF A MEDICAL PRACTITIONER AS AN EXPERT WITNESS

Forensic Science For Justice

TRUTH IN COURT – DUTY OF THE EXPERT, SERVICE TO JUSTICE

1. INTRODUCTION

The Court is a place of justice where evidence is recorded, evaluated and used to reach the truth. A Medical Practitioner, when called to court as an Expert Witness, has a duty to assist the court with his specialized knowledge impartially, honestly and responsibly.

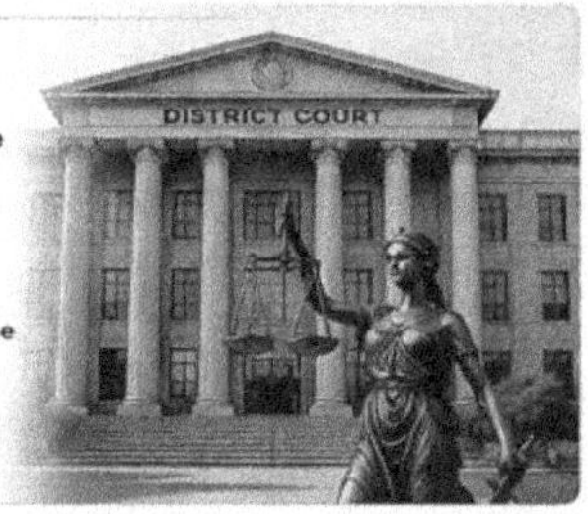

2. ROLE OF MEDICAL PRACTITIONER AS EXPERT WITNESS

- To provide independent and unbiased medical opinion.
- To explain scientific facts in simple and clear language.
- To help the court understand medical evidence.
- To answer questions based on knowledge and experience.
- To maintain professionalism and dignity of the medical profession.

3. COURT PROCEDURE – STEP BY STEP

1. **Filing of Complaint / FIR** – The process begins when a complaint is filed or an FIR is registered with the police.
2. **Investigation** – Police investigate the case, collect evidence and send the accused for medical examination if required.
3. **Medical Examination** – The doctor examines the victim/accused and prepares the medical report.
4. **Charge Sheet** – Police file charge sheet in the court against the accused.
5. **Framing of Charges** – The court considers the charge sheet and frames charges against the accused.
6. **Prosecution Evidence** – Prosecution presents witnesses and documents to prove the case.
7. **Expert Witness Examination** – The medical practitioner is called as an expert witness to present his opinion.
8. **Defense Evidence** – Defense may cross-examine prosecution witnesses and present their evidence.
9. **Arguments** – Both sides present final arguments before the court.
10. **Judgment** – The court evaluates all evidence and delivers the judgment.
11. **Order / Sentence** – If the accused is found guilty, the court passes the appropriate order or sentence.

4. CONDUCT OF MEDICAL PRACTITIONER AS EXPERT WITNESS

- Be punctual and dress formally.
- Carry all relevant documents, reports and summons.
- Take an oath to speak the truth and only the truth.
- Give clear, concise and truthful answers.
- Do not guess or give opinions beyond your expertise.
- Maintain calm, respect and patience during questioning.
- Do not argue with the lawyer; answer only what is asked.
- Do not disclose patient's identity unnecessarily.
- Your duty is to the court, not to the party who called you.
- Do not express personal bias or opinion.

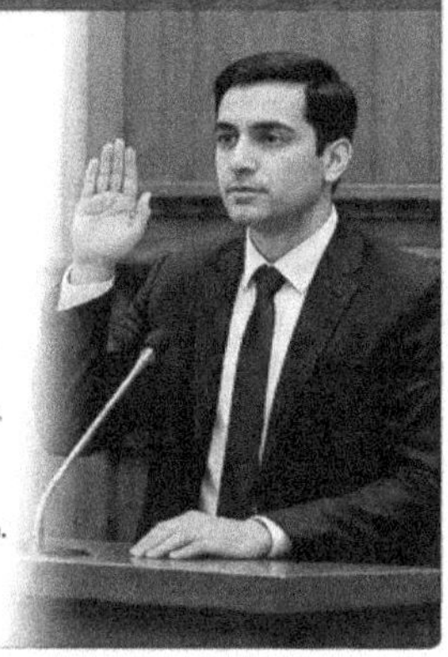

5. TYPES OF QUESTIONS IN COURT

Examination-in-Chief (By the lawyer who called you)	Cross-Examination (By the opposite lawyer)
✓ Establish facts.	Test credibility.
✓ Elicit information.	Challenge accuracy.
✓ Open-ended questions.	Leading questions.
✓ Non-leading questions.	May try to confuse.

Answer clearly, briefly and truthfully. If you do not know – say "I do not know".

6. DO's AND DON'Ts FOR EXPERT WITNESS

DO's	DON'Ts
Tell the truth.	Do not argue or show anger.
Be calm and confident.	Do not volunteer information.
Listen carefully to each question.	Do not guess or make assumptions.
Answer in your own words.	Do not use medical terms unnecessarily.
Refer to your notes if allowed.	Do not discuss the case outside the court.
Maintain professional ethics.	

7. RIGHTS OF AN EXPERT WITNESS

- To receive reasonable fee and conveyance.
- To be treated with respect in the court.
- To seek clarification if needed.
- To be protected from harassment or intimidation.
- To maintain confidentiality of records.

8. RESPONSIBILITIES OF AN EXPERT WITNESS

- Duty to the court and justice.
- Provide unbiased opinion.
- Use scientific knowledge and experience.
- Record findings accurately and honestly.
- Uphold dignity of medical profession.

7. 9. FLOW CHART – EXPERT WITNESS IN COURT

Receive Summons → Prepare & Review Documents → Appear in Court (Punctuality) → Take Oath → Examination-in-Chief → Cross-Examination → Re-Examination (if any) → Thank the Court & Leave

For Learning Resources & Educational Videos

Visha Vaidya

Dr Anil Kumar Y
Assistant Professor
Department of Agada Tantra (Visha Chikitsa OPD)
TMAE's Ayurveda Medical College & Hospital, Hospete

"Justice is truth in action, and truth is the duty of an expert."

PRACTICAL NO. 15

FIELD VISIT REPORT

VISIT TO COURT – OBSERVATION OF COURT PROCEDURE AND CONDUCT OF A MEDICAL PRACTITIONER AS AN EXPERT WITNESS

(Mandatory Practical Activity)

Date of Visit: __________

Name of Court: ______________________

Place: ______________________

Faculty Accompanying: ______________________

1. Title of Visit

Visit to Court for Observation of Court Procedure and Conduct of a Medical Practitioner as an Expert Witness.

2. Objectives

1. To understand the structure and functioning of a court.
2. To observe judicial proceedings.
3. To study the role of a medical practitioner as an expert witness.
4. To understand examination and cross-examination procedures.

3. Introduction

Courts play an important role in the administration of justice. Medical practitioners may be summoned to court as expert witnesses to provide scientific and professional opinions regarding medico-legal cases. Their evidence assists the court in reaching fair conclusions.

4. Observations

A. General Information

- Name of Court: ____________________
- Type of Court: Civil / Criminal / Sessions Court
- Date of Visit: ____________________
- Presiding Judge: ____________________

B. Court Procedure Observed

Sl. No.	Procedure	Observation
1	Calling of Cases	Cases called according to the cause list
2	Appearance of Parties	Presence of advocates, accused and witnesses
3	Recording of Evidence	Statements recorded under oath
4	Examination-in-Chief	Witness examined by the party calling the witness
5	Cross-Examination	Witness questioned by the opposite party
6	Re-examination	Clarification of evidence if required
7	Arguments	Presentation of legal arguments
8	Judgment/Order	Pronouncement by the court

C. Role of Medical Practitioner as Expert Witness

Duties Observed

- Appears before court when summoned.
- Takes oath before giving evidence.
- Produces medical records when required.
- Explains medical findings clearly and scientifically.
- Gives impartial expert opinion.
- Answers questions during examination and cross-examination.

D. Conduct of Expert Witness

Expected Conduct	Observation
Punctual appearance before court	__________
Proper professional attire	__________
Respectful behaviour towards court	__________
Clear and unbiased testimony	__________
Reliance on medical records and facts	__________
Maintenance of confidentiality	__________

5. Important Documents Observed

- Medico-Legal Case (MLC) Records
- Injury Reports
- Postmortem Reports
- Expert Medical Opinions
- Laboratory Reports

6. Learning Outcomes

1. Understood the basic court procedure.
2. Observed recording of evidence and witness examination.
3. Learned the role and responsibilities of an expert witness.
4. Understood the importance of accurate medical documentation.
5. Appreciated the ethical and legal duties of medical practitioners in courts.

7. Conclusion

The court visit provided practical exposure to judicial proceedings and the role of a medical practitioner as an expert witness. Accurate medical records, scientific opinion and professional conduct are essential for assisting the court in the administration of justice.

8. Result

Observed the court procedure, including examination of witnesses and judicial proceedings, and understood the conduct, responsibilities and significance of a medical practitioner serving as an expert witness.

Teacher's Signature

Student's Signature

PRACTICAL NO. 15

FIELD VISIT REPORT

VISIT TO MORTUARY FOR OBSERVATION OF MEDICO-LEGAL AUTOPSY

Date of Visit: __________

Place of Visit: _______________________

Name of Hospital/Mortuary: _______________________

Faculty Accompanying: _______________________

1. Title of Visit

Visit to Mortuary for Observation of Medico-Legal Autopsy Procedure.

2. Objectives

1. To observe the procedure of medico-legal autopsy.
2. To understand the medico-legal importance of postmortem examination.
3. To study external and internal examination of a dead body.
4. To observe preservation of viscera and preparation of autopsy reports.

3. Introduction

A medico-legal autopsy is a scientific examination of a dead body conducted under legal authority to determine the cause, manner and time of death. It also helps identify injuries, poisoning, disease and other medico-legal aspects relevant to investigation and administration of justice.

4. Observations

A. General Information

- Postmortem Number: ____________________
- Date & Time of Autopsy: ____________________
- Age/Sex of Deceased: ____________________
- Conducted By: ____________________
- Police Station: ____________________

B. Procedure Observed

1. Identification of the Body

- Verification of identity by relatives/police.
- Examination of documents and requisition letter.

2. External Examination

- Recording age, sex, height and built.
- Examination of clothing and personal belongings.
- Documentation of identification marks.
- Observation of postmortem changes:
    - Rigor mortis
    - Postmortem lividity
    - Decomposition changes
- Examination and measurement of injuries.

3. Internal Examination

Head and Brain

- Scalp reflected.
- Skull opened.
- Brain examined for injuries and abnormalities.

Thorax

- Chest cavity opened.
- Heart and lungs examined.

Abdomen

- Abdominal cavity opened.
- Liver, spleen, kidneys and gastrointestinal tract examined.

4. Collection and Preservation of Samples

- Stomach and its contents.
- Small intestine and contents.
- Liver sample.
- Kidney sample.
- Blood and urine (if required).

5. Documentation

- Findings recorded systematically.
- Cause of death assessed.
- Autopsy report prepared.

C. Findings Observed

Examination	Observation
Identification Marks	____________________
Postmortem Changes	____________________
External Injuries	____________________
Internal Findings	____________________
Viscera Preserved	____________________
Probable Cause of Death	____________________

5. Medico-Legal Importance of Autopsy

1. Establishes cause of death.
2. Helps determine manner of death (natural, accidental, suicidal or homicidal).
3. Assists criminal investigations.
4. Identifies poisoning and other pathological conditions.
5. Provides evidence for courts of law.

6. Learning Outcomes

1. Understood the sequence of medico-legal autopsy.
2. Observed external and internal examination procedures.
3. Learned the importance of documenting injuries.
4. Observed viscera preservation techniques.
5. Understood the medico-legal significance of autopsy findings.

7. Conclusion

The mortuary visit provided practical exposure to medico-legal autopsy procedures, including identification of the body, external and internal examinations, collection of specimens and preparation of autopsy reports. The autopsy plays a crucial role in determining the cause and manner of death.

8. Result

Observed the medico-legal autopsy procedure and understood the systematic examination of the body, documentation of findings, preservation of viscera and formulation of opinion regarding the cause of death.

Teacher's Signature

Student's Signature

VISIT TO SNAKE PARK

Observe Live Specimens of Snake

Visha Chikitsa OPD

Forensic Science For Justice

KNOW SNAKES – RESPECT NATURE – PREVENT SNAKEBITE – SAVE LIVES

1. OBJECTIVES OF THE VISIT

- To observe live specimens of snakes.
- To understand the diversity and
- identification of venomous and non-venomous snakes.
- To study the behavior, habitat and adaptations of snakes.
- To create awareness about snakebite prevention and conservation.
- To learn about venom extraction and its uses.

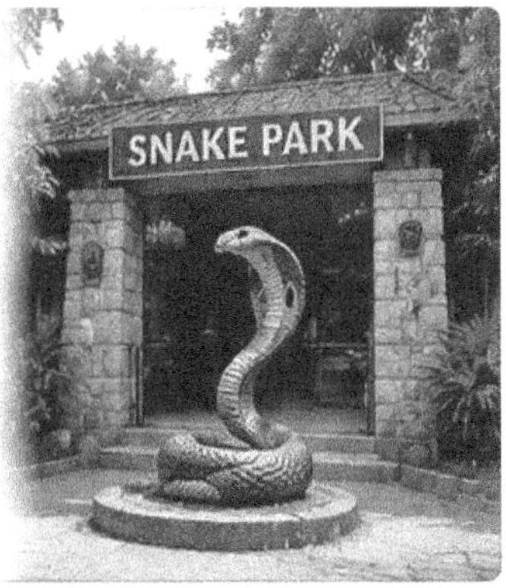

2. WHAT IS A SNAKE PARK?

A Snake Park is a specialized facility where live snakes are housed in naturalistic environments for education, research, conservation and venom collection.

- Education & Awareness
- Research & Conservation
- Venom Collection
- Public Safety & Conservation

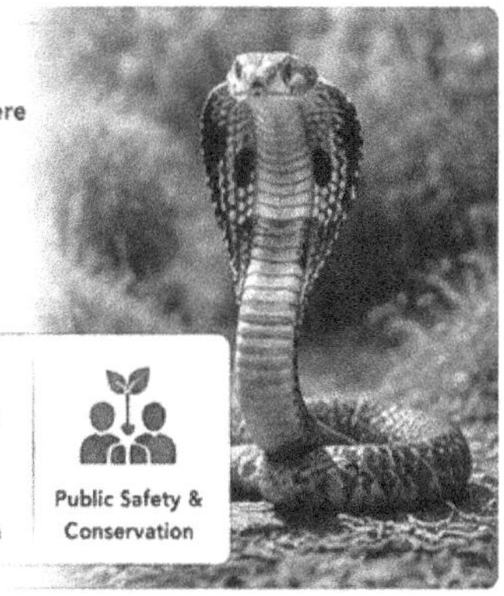

3. COMMON SNAKES OBSERVED IN SNAKE PARK

VENOMOUS SNAKES

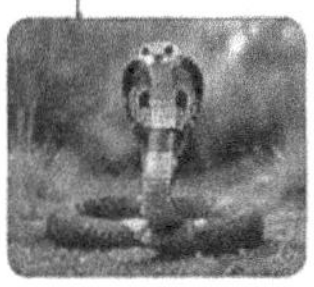
Indian Cobra (*Naja naja*)

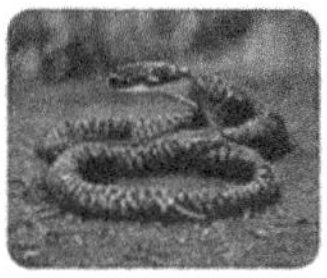
Common Krait (*Bungarus caeruleus*)

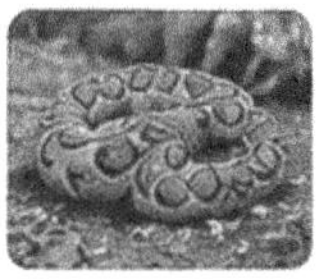
Russell's Viper (*Daboia russelii*)

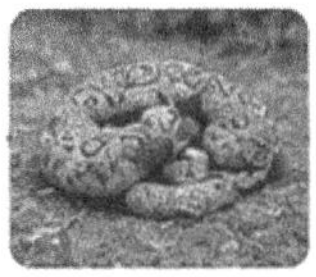
Saw-scaled Viper (*Echis carinatus*)

NON-VENOMOUS SNAKES

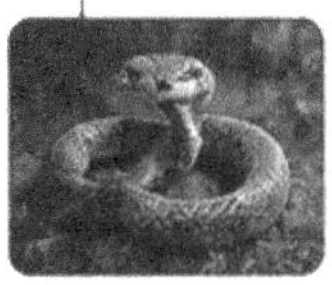
Rat Snake (*Ptyas mucosa*)

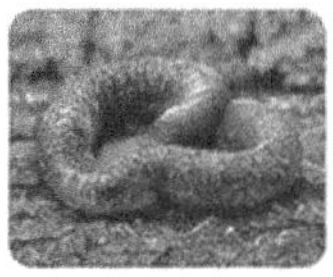
Common Sand Boa (*Eryx conicus*)

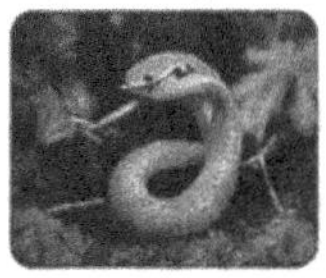
Bronze Back Tree Snake (*Dendrelaphis tristis*)

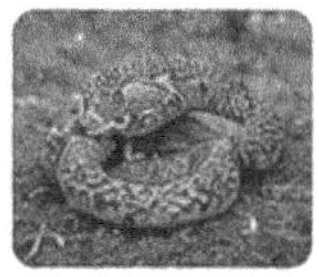
Checkered Keelback (*Fowlea piscator*)

4. WHAT WE OBSERVE

- Morphology of snakes – head, scales, eyes, tail.
- Identification of venomous vs non-venomous snakes.
- Behavior and defensive mechanisms.
- Habitat & ecological role of snakes.
- Breeding and life cycle.
- Snake rescue and handling techniques (demonstration).

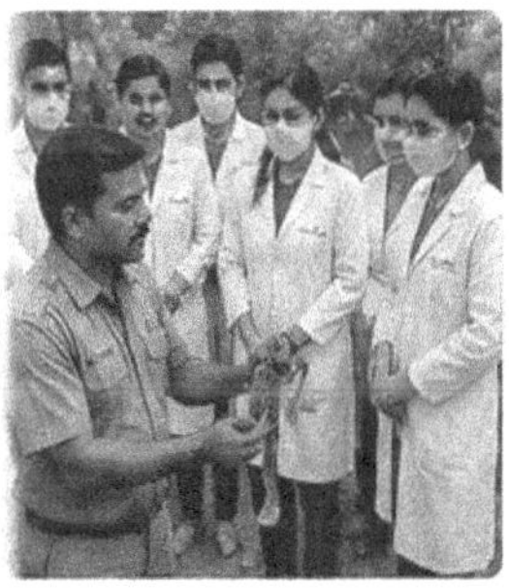

5. LIVE DEMONSTRATION & LEARNING

- Safe handling of live specimens (by trained experts only).
- Venom extraction process (demonstration).
- Display of snake anatomy – fangs, venom glands, scales.
- First aid and do's & don'ts in snakebite.

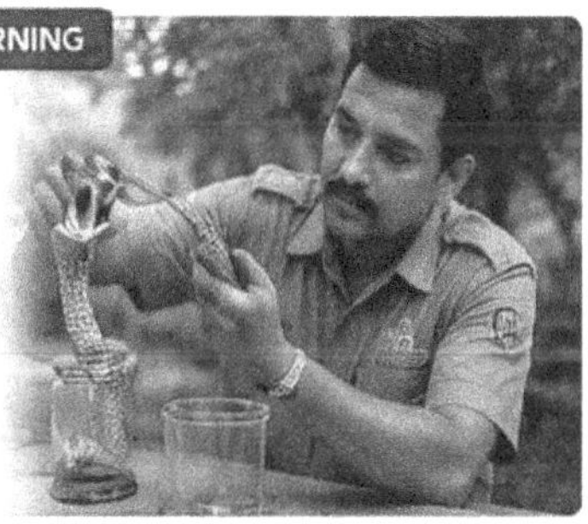

6. DO'S AND DON'TS IN SNAKE ENCOUNTER

DO'S	DON'TS
Stay calm and move away slowly.	Do not try to kill or capture.
Keep a safe distance.	Do not disturb or tease snakes.
Wear protective footwear.	Do not apply cuts, suction or tourniquets.
Use a torch at night.	Do not give alcohol or food to the victim.
Seek medical help immediately in case of bite.	

7. IMPORTANCE OF SNAKE PARK

- Helps in conservation of snake species.
- Supports research in toxinology and pharmacology.
- Provides antivenom for saving lives.
- Educates the public and reduces snake fear & killing.
- Promotes ecological balance.

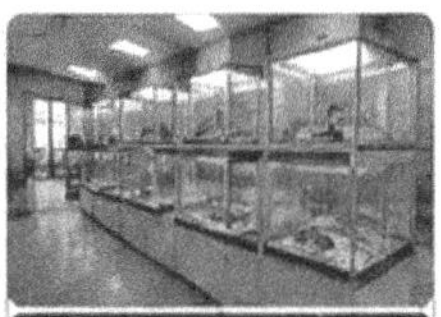

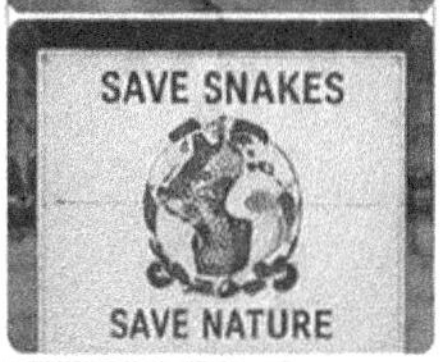

8. KEY TAKEAWAY

"Snakes are not our enemy, they are protectors of nature. Let us learn, respect and live in harmony with them."

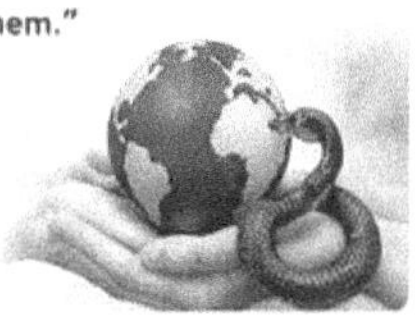

OBSERVATION RECORD

- Date of Visit ....
- Place ....
- Snakes Observed ....
- Learning Outcome ....

SCAN TO LEARN MORE

REMEMBER

"A little knowledge can save a life."
Awareness today – Safety tomorrow."

Dr Anil Kumar Y
Assistant Professor
Department of Agada Tantra
(Visha Chikitsa OPD)
TMAE's Ayurveda Medical College & Hospital
Hospete, Karnataka

Visha Vaidya

BE AWARE – BE PREPARED – BE SAFE

PRACTICAL NO. 15

FIELD VISIT REPORT

VISIT TO SNAKE PARK – OBSERVATION OF LIVE SPECIMENS OF SNAKES

(Mandatory Practical Activity)

Date of Visit: __________

Place of Visit: ______________________

Name of Snake Park: ______________________

Faculty Accompanying: ______________________

1. Title of Visit

Visit to Snake Park for Observation of Live Specimens of Snakes.

2. Objectives

1. To observe live specimens of poisonous and non-poisonous snakes.
2. To identify distinguishing features of various snake species.
3. To understand the medico-toxicological importance of snake envenomation.
4. To learn preventive measures against snakebite.

---

3. Introduction

Snakebite is an important medical emergency and a significant public health problem in India. Observation of live snakes helps in identification of species, understanding their behaviour and recognizing poisonous snakes commonly encountered in medico-toxicological practice.

4. Observations

A. General Information

- Name of Snake Park: __________________
- Location: __________________
- Date of Visit: __________________

- Number of Species Observed: ____________________

B. Live Specimens Observed

Sl. No.	Common Name	Scientific Name	Poisonous/Non-Poisonous	Important Features
1	Indian Cobra	Naja naja	Poisonous	Hood with spectacle mark
2	Common Krait	Bungarus caeruleus	Poisonous	Glossy black body with white bands
3	Russell's Viper	Daboia russelii	Poisonous	Chain-like spots on body
4	Saw-scaled Viper	Echis carinatus	Poisonous	Rough scales and zig-zag movement
5	Rat Snake	Ptyas mucosa	Non-poisonous	Long slender body
6	Indian Rock Python	Python molurus	Non-poisonous	Large constrictor snake

C. Identification Features Observed

Poisonous Snakes

- Presence of venom apparatus.
- Distinctive body markings.
- Characteristic head and fang structure.
- Behavioural characteristics.

Non-Poisonous Snakes

- Absence of venom glands.
- Different dentition pattern.
- Generally harmless to humans.

D. Information Obtained During Visit

1. Habitat and distribution of snakes.
2. Feeding habits and behaviour.
3. Identification of venomous snakes.
4. Prevention of snakebite.

5. First aid measures in snakebite.
6. Importance of anti-snake venom (ASV).

5. Medico-Toxicological Importance

Snake Group	Type of Venom	Major Effects
Cobra	Neurotoxic	Paralysis, respiratory failure
Krait	Neurotoxic	Neuromuscular paralysis
Russell's Viper	Hemotoxic/Vasculotoxic	Bleeding disorders, shock
Saw-scaled Viper	Hemotoxic/Vasculotoxic	Hemorrhage and coagulopathy

6. Snakebite First Aid Observed

- Reassure the patient.
- Immobilize the bitten limb.
- Avoid incision, suction and tourniquets.
- Transport patient immediately to hospital.
- Administer Anti-Snake Venom (ASV) when indicated.

7. Learning Outcomes

1. Observed live specimens of common snakes.
2. Learned distinguishing features of poisonous and non-poisonous snakes.
3. Understood the clinical importance of snake envenomation.
4. Learned preventive measures and first aid in snakebite.
5. Appreciated the role of snake conservation and public awareness.

8. Conclusion

The visit to the Snake Park provided practical exposure to the identification of common snake species, their behaviour, venom characteristics and medico-toxicological significance. It enhanced understanding of snakebite prevention and management.

9. Result

Observed live specimens of poisonous and non-poisonous snakes and understood their identification, venom characteristics, medico-toxicological importance and basic principles of snakebite management.

Teacher's Signature

Student's Signature

Visha Chikitsa OPD

VISIT TO CASUALITY

WATCH THE PROCEDURE OF RESUSCITATION AND EMERGENCY MANAGEMENT

Forensic Science For Justice

EVERY SECOND COUNTS – BE PREPARED, BE SKILLED, SAVE LIVES

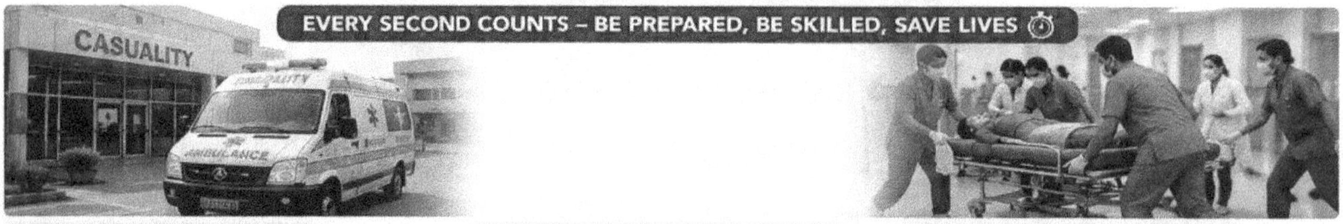

1. OBJECTIVES OF THE VISIT

- To observe the working of casualty / emergency department.
- To understand the triage process and priority of care.
- To watch the procedure of resuscitation (CPR, BLS, ACLS)
- To learn emergency management of medical and surgical cases.
- To understand the use of emergency drugs and equipment.

2. CASUALITY DEPARTMENT – OVERVIEW

The Casuality Department is the first point of contact for any emergency patient. It provides immediate care and stabilization to save life, prevent further deterioration and prepare the patient for definitive treatment.

3. TRIAGE – PRIORITY OF CARE

RED	IMMEDIATE	Life threatening – Needs immediate attention
YELLOW	DELAYED	Serious but stable – Can wait
GREEN	MINOR	Stable – Minimal treatment
BLACK	EXPECTANT	Not survivable – Palliative care

4. PROCEDURE OF RESUSCITATION – BLS (BASIC LIFE SUPPORT)

1. **ASSESS** Check response and call for help
2. **AIRWAY** Open airway (Head tilt – Chin lift)
3. **BREATHING** Look, listen and feel for breathing
4. **CIRCULATION** Check pulse Start CPR if no pulse
5. **CPR** 30 compressions : 2 breaths (Adult)
6. **AED** Attach AED as soon as available
7. **CONTINUE** Continue until help arrives or patient recovers

CHAIN OF SURVIVAL

Early Recognition → Early CPR → Early Defibrillation → Advanced Care → Post Resuscitation Care

5. ADVANCED LIFE SUPPORT (ACLS)

- ✓ Continuous assessment (ABCD approach)
- ✓ Airway with advanced devices
- ✓ Oxygenation and ventilation
- ✓ ECG monitoring
- ✓ Defibrillation for shockable rhythms
- ✓ Emergency drugs administration
- ✓ Treat reversible causes (H's & T's)
  - Hypoxia
  - Hypovolemia
  - Hydrogen ion (Acidosis)
  - Hypo/Hyperkalemia
  - Hypothermia
  - Tension pneumothorax
  - Tamponade
  - Toxins
  - Thrombosis

6. EMERGENCY MANAGEMENT – COMMON CONDITIONS

- **CARDIAC ARREST** CPR, Defibrillation, Drugs, Airway, Monitoring
- **SHOCK** Fluids, Oxygen, Blood, Treat cause
- **ACUTE ASTHMA** Oxygen, Nebulization, Bronchodilators
- **STROKE** Time critical management, Thrombolysis (if eligible)
- **TRAUMA** Airway, Breathing, Circulation, Disability, Exposure (ABCDE)
- **POISONING** Decontamination, Antidotes, Supportive care
- **DIABETIC EMERGENCY** Check RBS, Fluids, Insulin as per protocol
- **SEIZURE** Protect airway, Control fits, Treat cause

7. EMERGENCY EQUIPMENTS OBSERVED

Defibrillator, Cardiac Monitor, Ambu Bag, Suction Apparatus, Oxygen Cylinder, Airway Devices, Crash Cart, Spine Board, Emergency Drugs

8. EMERGENCY DRUGS COMMONLY USED

- ✓ Adrenaline
- ✓ Atropine
- ✓ Amiodarone
- ✓ Aspirin
- ✓ Nitroglycerin
- ✓ Salbutamol
- ✓ Hydrocortisone
- ✓ Magnesium Sulphate
- ✓ Diazepam
- ✓ Dopamine / Noradrenaline
- ✓ Others as per protocol

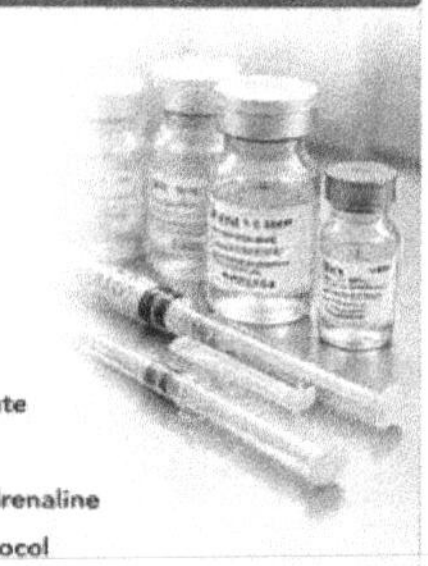

9. PROCEDURE FLOW IN CASUALITY

Patient Arrival → Triage → Initial Assessment → Stabilization & Resuscitation → Investigation → Definitive Treatment / Referral

10. LEARNING OUTCOMES OF THE VISIT

- Gained knowledge about emergency workflow.
- Understood importance of time and teamwork.
- Observed and appreciated life saving procedures.
- Learned the practical use of emergency equipment and drugs.
- Realized the responsibility and role of medical professionals in

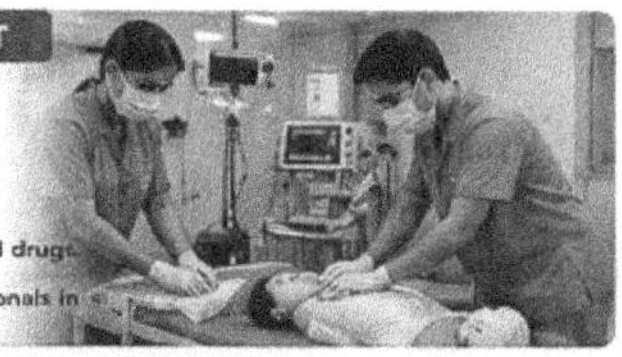

DO'S AND DON'TS IN EMERGENCY AREA

DO'S

- Stay calm and act quickly.
- Follow standard protocols.
- Ensure patient safety.
- Maintain aseptic precautions.
- Communicate clearly.
- Document accurately.

DON'TS

- Do not panic or crowd around.
- Do not delay essential care.
- Do not use mobile phones unnecessarily.
- Do not give wrong information.
- Do not leave equipment unattended.

NOTE

Emergency care saves lives. Your knowledge, skills and presence of mind can make the difference between life and death.

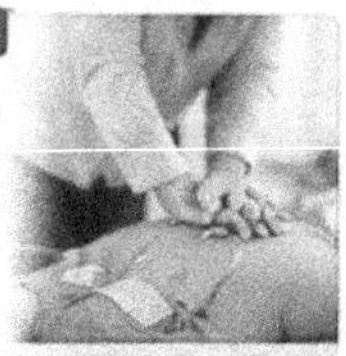

REMEMBER

"In emergencies, we do not rise to the level of our expectations, we fall to the level of our training."

Scan for Emergency Care Guidelines & Videos

Visha Vaidya

Dr Anil Kumar Y
Assistant Professor
Department of Agada Tantra (Visha Chikitsa OPD)
TMAE's Ayurveda Medical College & Hospital, Hospete

"Be prepared. Save a life." You may be the reason someone lives today."

PRACTICAL NO. 15

FIELD VISIT REPORT

VISIT TO CASUALTY (EMERGENCY DEPARTMENT)

OBSERVATION OF RESUSCITATION AND EMERGENCY MANAGEMENT

(Mandatory Practical Activity)

Date of Visit: __________

Hospital: ______________________

Faculty Accompanying: ______________________

1. Title of Visit

Visit to Casualty/Emergency Department for Observation of Resuscitation and Emergency Management.

2. Objectives

1. To observe the functioning of the Casualty Department.
2. To understand the principles of emergency patient management.
3. To observe resuscitation procedures.
4. To learn the role of healthcare professionals during emergencies.

3. Introduction

The Casualty or Emergency Department provides immediate medical care to critically ill and injured patients. Rapid assessment, resuscitation and stabilization are essential to save life and prevent complications.

4. Observations

A. General Information

- Name of Hospital: ____________________
- Date of Visit: ____________________
- Casualty In-charge: ____________________

B. Emergency Cases Commonly Seen

Sl. No.	Emergency Condition
1	Road Traffic Accidents
2	Poisoning Cases
3	Snake Bite Cases
4	Burns
5	Cardiac Emergencies
6	Respiratory Distress
7	Trauma Cases
8	Unconscious Patients

C. Resuscitation Procedure Observed

Primary Survey (ABCDE Approach)

Step	Observation
A	Airway assessment and maintenance
B	Breathing assessment and oxygen administration
C	Circulation assessment, pulse and blood pressure monitoring
D	Disability assessment (neurological status)
E	Exposure and complete examination

Emergency Measures Observed

- Airway maintenance.
- Oxygen therapy.
- Intravenous fluid administration.
- Monitoring of vital signs.
- Cardiopulmonary Resuscitation (CPR) when indicated.
- Wound care and bleeding control.
- Emergency drug administration.

D. Equipment Observed

Sl. No.	Equipment	Purpose
1	Oxygen Cylinder	Oxygen delivery
2	Ambu Bag	Assisted ventilation
3	Defibrillator	Cardiac resuscitation
4	Suction Apparatus	Airway clearance
5	Cardiac Monitor	Monitoring vital parameters
6	Pulse Oximeter	Monitoring oxygen saturation
7	Emergency Drug Trolley	Emergency medications
8	Ventilator	Mechanical ventilation

E. Healthcare Team Observed

- Casualty Medical Officer
- Emergency Physician
- Nursing Staff
- Laboratory Personnel
- Support Staff

5. Learning Outcomes

1. Understood the organization of the Emergency Department.
2. Observed the ABCDE approach in emergency management.
3. Learned basic principles of resuscitation.
4. Understood the importance of teamwork during emergencies.
5. Observed life-saving equipment and procedures.

6. Conclusion

The visit to the Casualty Department provided practical exposure to emergency care, resuscitation techniques and patient stabilization procedures. Prompt assessment and management are essential for improving patient outcomes in emergencies.

7. Result

Observed the procedures of resuscitation and emergency management in the Casualty Department, including airway management, oxygen therapy, monitoring, intravenous access and basic life-support measures.

Teacher's Signature

Student's Signature

PRACTICAL NO. 15

FIELD VISIT REPORT

VISIT TO OCCUPATIONAL HAZARDS CENTRE

OBSERVATION OF TYPES AND MANAGEMENT OF OCCUPATIONAL HAZARD CASES

Date of Visit: __________

Place of Visit: ______________________

Name of Occupational Health Centre: ______________________

Faculty Accompanying: ______________________

1. Title of Visit

Visit to Occupational Hazards Centre for Observation of Types and Management of Occupational Hazard Cases.

2. Objectives

1. To understand occupational hazards and occupational diseases.
2. To observe different types of occupational hazard cases.
3. To study preventive and management measures.
4. To understand the role of occupational health services in worker safety.

3. Introduction

Occupational hazards are health risks arising from exposure to harmful physical, chemical, biological, ergonomic or psychosocial factors at the workplace. Occupational health centres provide preventive, diagnostic and rehabilitative services to workers exposed to such hazards.

4. Observations

A. General Information

- Name of Centre: ____________________
- Location: ____________________
- Type of Industry/Workers Covered: ____________________
- Date of Visit: ____________________

B. Types of Occupational Hazards Observed

Sl. No.	Hazard Type	Examples
1	Physical Hazards	Noise, heat, radiation, vibration
2	Chemical Hazards	Pesticides, solvents, heavy metals, toxic gases
3	Biological Hazards	Bacteria, viruses, fungi
4	Mechanical Hazards	Machinery injuries, cuts, crush injuries
5	Ergonomic Hazards	Repetitive strain injuries, back pain
6	Psychosocial Hazards	Stress, anxiety, workplace burnout

C. Occupational Diseases/Cases Observed

Sl. No.	Disease/Condition	Associated Occupation
1	Silicosis	Mining, stone cutting
2	Asbestosis	Asbestos industry
3	Noise-Induced Hearing Loss	Factory workers
4	Pesticide Poisoning	Agricultural workers
5	Contact Dermatitis	Chemical industry workers
6	Occupational Asthma	Dust and chemical exposure workers
7	Musculoskeletal Disorders	Manual labourers, office workers
8	Heat Stress	Foundry and outdoor workers

D. Management Observed

1. Clinical Assessment

- Occupational history taking.
- Exposure assessment.
- Physical examination.
- Laboratory investigations.

2. Treatment

- Symptomatic management.
- Removal from exposure.
- Emergency care where required.
- Specific therapy according to condition.

3. Preventive Measures

- Use of Personal Protective Equipment (PPE).
- Workplace safety education.
- Periodic health check-ups.
- Environmental monitoring.

4. Rehabilitation

- Physiotherapy.
- Occupational counselling.
- Return-to-work assessment.
- Long-term follow-up.

E. Safety Equipment Observed

Equipment	Purpose
Safety Helmet	Head protection
Safety Goggles	Eye protection
Face Mask/Respirator	Respiratory protection
Ear Plugs	Hearing protection
Protective Gloves	Hand protection
Safety Shoes	Foot protection

Equipment	Purpose
Protective Clothing	Body protection

5. Learning Outcomes

1. Understood various occupational hazards and diseases.
2. Observed methods of diagnosis and management.
3. Learned the importance of occupational history.
4. Understood preventive measures and use of PPE.
5. Appreciated the role of occupational health services in worker welfare.

6. Conclusion

The visit provided practical exposure to occupational hazards, occupational diseases and their management. Proper preventive measures, workplace safety practices and periodic health surveillance are essential for protecting workers' health.

7. Result

Observed different types of occupational hazard cases and understood their diagnosis, treatment, preventive measures and rehabilitation services provided through occupational health centres.

Teacher's Signature

Student's Signature

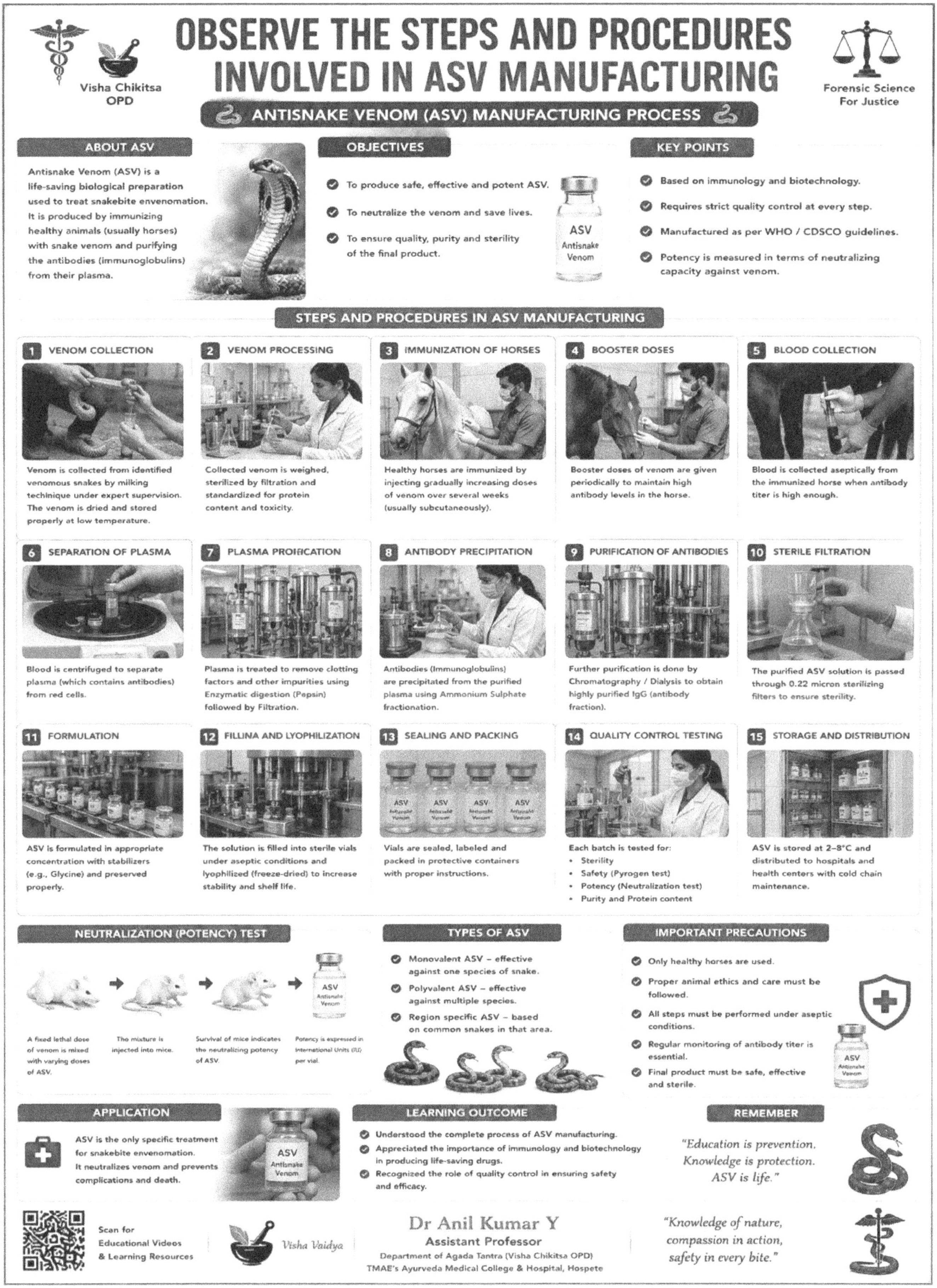

Visha Chikitsa OPD
OBSERVE THE STEPS AND PROCEDURES INVOLVED IN ASV MANUFACTURING
Forensic Science For Justice
ANTISNAKE VENOM (ASV) MANUFACTURING PROCESS
ABOUT ASV
Antisnake Venom (ASV) is a life-saving biological preparation used to treat snakebite envenomation. It is produced by immunizing healthy animals (usually horses) with snake venom and purifying the antibodies (immunoglobulins) from their plasma.
OBJECTIVES
To produce safe, effective and potent ASV.
To neutralize the venom and save lives.
To ensure quality, purity and sterility of the final product.
ASV Antisnake Venom
KEY POINTS
Based on immunology and biotechnology.
Requires strict quality control at every step.
Manufactured as per WHO / CDSCO guidelines.
Potency is measured in terms of neutralizing capacity against venom.
STEPS AND PROCEDURES IN ASV MANUFACTURING
1 VENOM COLLECTION
Venom is collected from identified venomous snakes by milking techinique under expert supervision. The venom is dried and stored properly at low temperature.
2 VENOM PROCESSING
Collected venom is weighed, sterilized by filtration and standardized for protein content and toxicity.
3 IMMUNIZATION OF HORSES
Healthy horses are immunized by injecting gradually increasing doses of venom over several weeks (usually subcutaneously).
4 BOOSTER DOSES
Booster doses of venom are given periodically to maintain high antibody levels in the horse.
5 BLOOD COLLECTION
Blood is collected aseptically from the immunized horse when antibody titer is high enough.
6 SEPARATION OF PLASMA
Blood is centrifuged to separate plasma (which contains antibodies) from red cells.
7 PLASMA PROIFICATION
Plasma is treated to remove clotting factors and other impurities using Enzymatic digestion (Pepsin) followed by Filtration.
8 ANTIBODY PRECIPITATION
Antibodies (Immunoglobulins) are precipitated from the purified plasma using Ammonium Sulphate fractionation.
9 PURIFICATION OF ANTIBODIES
Further purification is done by Chromatography / Dialysis to obtain highly purified IgG (antibody fraction).
10 STERILE FILTRATION
The purified ASV solution is passed through 0.22 micron sterilizing filters to ensure sterility.
11 FORMULATION
ASV is formulated in appropriate concentration with stabilizers (e.g., Glycine) and preserved properly.
12 FILLINA AND LYOPHILIZATION
The solution is filled into sterile vials under aseptic conditions and lyophilized (freeze-dried) to increase stability and shelf life.
13 SEALING AND PACKING
Vials are sealed, labeled and packed in protective containers with proper instructions.
14 QUALITY CONTROL TESTING
Each batch is tested for:
• Sterility
• Safety (Pyrogen test)
• Potency (Neutralization test)
• Purity and Protein content
15 STORAGE AND DISTRIBUTION
ASV is stored at 2–8°C and distributed to hospitals and health centers with cold chain maintenance.
NEUTRALIZATION (POTENCY) TEST
A fixed lethal dose of venom is mixed with varying doses of ASV.
The mixture is injected into mice.
Survival of mice indicates the neutralizing potency of ASV.
Potency is expressed in International Units (IU) per vial.
TYPES OF ASV
Monovalent ASV – effective against one species of snake.
Polyvalent ASV – effective against multiple species.
Region specific ASV – based on common snakes in that area.
IMPORTANT PRECAUTIONS
Only healthy horses are used.
Proper animal ethics and care must be followed.
All steps must be performed under aseptic conditions.
Regular monitoring of antibody titer is essential.
Final product must be safe, effective and sterile.
APPLICATION
ASV is the only specific treatment for snakebite envenomation.
It neutralizes venom and prevents complications and death.
LEARNING OUTCOME
Understood the complete process of ASV manufacturing.
Appreciated the importance of immunology and biotechnology in producing life-saving drugs.
Recognized the role of quality control in ensuring safety and efficacy.
REMEMBER
"Education is prevention. Knowledge is protection. ASV is life."
Scan for Educational Videos & Learning Resources
Visha Vaidya
Dr Anil Kumar Y
Assistant Professor
Department of Agada Tantra (Visha Chikitsa OPD)
TMAE's Ayurveda Medical College & Hospital, Hospete
"Knowledge of nature, compassion in action, safety in every bite."

PRACTICAL NO. 15

FIELD VISIT REPORT

VISIT TO ANTI-SNAKE VENOM (ASV) MANUFACTURING CENTRE

OBSERVATION OF STEPS AND PROCEDURES INVOLVED IN ASV MANUFACTURING

Date of Visit: __________

Place of Visit: ______________________

Name of ASV Manufacturing Centre: ______________________

Faculty Accompanying: ______________________

1. Title of Visit

Visit to Anti-Snake Venom (ASV) Manufacturing Centre for Observation of Manufacturing Procedures.

2. Objectives

1. To understand the process of Anti-Snake Venom production.
2. To observe the collection and processing of snake venom.
3. To study quality control measures in ASV manufacturing.
4. To understand the importance of ASV in snakebite management.

3. Introduction

Anti-Snake Venom (ASV) is a biological product used for the treatment of venomous snakebite. It is prepared by immunizing healthy animals (usually horses) with small quantities of snake venom and collecting antibodies produced against the venom. These antibodies are purified and processed into ASV for therapeutic use.

4. Observations

A. General Information

- Name of Manufacturing Centre: ____________________
- Location: ____________________
- Date of Visit: ____________________
- Supervising Officer: ____________________

B. Steps Observed in ASV Manufacturing

Sl. No.	Step	Observation
1	Venom Collection	Venom collected from venomous snakes under controlled conditions
2	Venom Processing	Venom filtered, measured and preserved
3	Preparation of Venom Mixture	Standardized venom mixture prepared
4	Immunization of Horses	Small doses of venom injected at intervals
5	Antibody Production	Horses develop antibodies against venom
6	Blood Collection	Blood collected from immunized horses
7	Plasma Separation	Plasma separated from blood
8	Antibody Purification	Immunoglobulins purified and processed
9	Sterilization and Filtration	Product sterilized and filtered
10	Quality Control Testing	Safety, potency and sterility tests performed
11	Packaging and Storage	ASV packed, labelled and stored

C. Snake Venoms Used

Common Venomous Snakes Included in Polyvalent ASV

Snake	Scientific Name	Type of Venom
Indian Cobra	Naja naja	Neurotoxic
Common Krait	Bungarus caeruleus	Neurotoxic
Russell's Viper	Daboia russelii	Hemotoxic/Vasculotoxic
Saw-scaled Viper	Echis carinatus	Hemotoxic/Vasculotoxic

D. Quality Control Measures Observed

- Sterility testing.
- Potency testing.
- Safety testing.
- Batch standardization.
- Proper cold-chain maintenance.
- Labeling and documentation.

E. Storage Conditions

- Refrigerated storage.
- Protection from direct sunlight.
- Maintenance of recommended temperature.
- Monitoring of expiry date.

5. Importance of ASV

1. Specific treatment for venomous snakebite.
2. Neutralizes circulating venom.
3. Prevents severe complications and death.
4. Essential medicine in emergency snakebite management.
5. Reduces morbidity and mortality associated with envenomation.

6. Learning Outcomes

1. Understood the basic principles of ASV production.
2. Observed venom collection and processing methods.
3. Learned the role of horse immunization in antibody production.
4. Understood quality control procedures.
5. Appreciated the importance of ASV in clinical toxicology.

7. Conclusion

The visit provided practical exposure to the manufacturing process of Anti-Snake Venom, including venom collection, immunization, plasma processing, purification and quality control. ASV remains the most important specific treatment for venomous snakebite.

8. Result

Observed the steps and procedures involved in Anti-Snake Venom manufacturing, including venom collection, immunization, antibody production, purification, quality testing and storage.

Teacher's Signature

Student's Signature

PRACTICAL NO. 15

FIELD VISIT REPORT

VISIT TO CANCER TREATMENT CENTRE

OBSERVATION OF DIAGNOSIS, TREATMENT AND MANAGEMENT OF CANCER PATIENTS

Date of Visit: ___________

Place of Visit: ________________________

Name of Cancer Treatment Centre: ________________________

Faculty Accompanying: ________________________

1. Title of Visit

Visit to Cancer Treatment Centre for Observation of Cancer Diagnosis, Treatment and Patient Management.

2. Objectives

1. To understand the functioning of a Cancer Treatment Centre.
2. To observe diagnostic procedures used in cancer detection.
3. To study various modalities of cancer treatment.
4. To understand supportive and palliative care services.

3. Introduction

Cancer is a disease characterized by uncontrolled growth and spread of abnormal cells. Cancer treatment centres provide comprehensive care including diagnosis, surgery, chemotherapy, radiotherapy, immunotherapy and palliative care. Early diagnosis and multidisciplinary management improve patient outcomes.

4. Observations

A. General Information

- Name of Centre: ____________________
- Location: ____________________
- Date of Visit: ____________________
- Type of Centre: Government / Private / Teaching Hospital

B. Departments Observed

Sl. No.	Department	Function
1	Medical Oncology	Chemotherapy and systemic treatment
2	Surgical Oncology	Surgical management of cancer
3	Radiation Oncology	Radiotherapy services
4	Pathology Department	Histopathological diagnosis
5	Radiology Department	Imaging and cancer staging
6	Palliative Care Unit	Symptom relief and supportive care

C. Diagnostic Procedures Observed

Procedure	Purpose
Clinical Examination	Initial assessment
Biopsy	Confirmation of diagnosis
Fine Needle Aspiration Cytology (FNAC)	Cytological diagnosis
CT Scan	Tumour evaluation and staging
MRI	Detailed imaging
PET Scan	Detection of spread of cancer
Histopathology	Microscopic confirmation

D. Treatment Modalities Observed

1. Surgery

- Removal of tumour.
- Curative or palliative procedures.

2. Chemotherapy

- Administration of anti-cancer drugs.
- Monitoring for adverse effects.

3. Radiotherapy

- Use of ionizing radiation to destroy cancer cells.

4. Immunotherapy / Targeted Therapy

- Specific treatment directed against cancer cells.

5. Palliative Care

- Pain management.
- Psychological support.
- End-of-life care when required.

E. Common Cancer Cases Observed

Cancer Type	Common Site
Breast Cancer	Breast
Oral Cancer	Oral cavity
Lung Cancer	Lungs
Cervical Cancer	Cervix
Colorectal Cancer	Colon and Rectum
Prostate Cancer	Prostate Gland

5. Multidisciplinary Team Observed

- Medical Oncologist
- Surgical Oncologist
- Radiation Oncologist
- Pathologist
- Radiologist
- Oncology Nurses
- Psychologist/Counsellor
- Palliative Care Specialist

6. Learning Outcomes

1. Understood the organization and functioning of a cancer treatment centre.
2. Observed diagnostic procedures used for cancer detection.
3. Learned different treatment modalities available for cancer.
4. Understood the importance of multidisciplinary care.
5. Appreciated the role of palliative and supportive care services.

7. Conclusion

The visit provided practical exposure to cancer diagnosis, treatment planning and patient management. Comprehensive care involving surgery, chemotherapy, radiotherapy and supportive care is essential for improving quality of life and treatment outcomes in cancer patients.

8. Result

Observed the functioning of a Cancer Treatment Centre, including diagnostic investigations, treatment modalities, patient counselling, supportive care and multidisciplinary management of cancer patients.

Teacher's Signature

Student's Signature

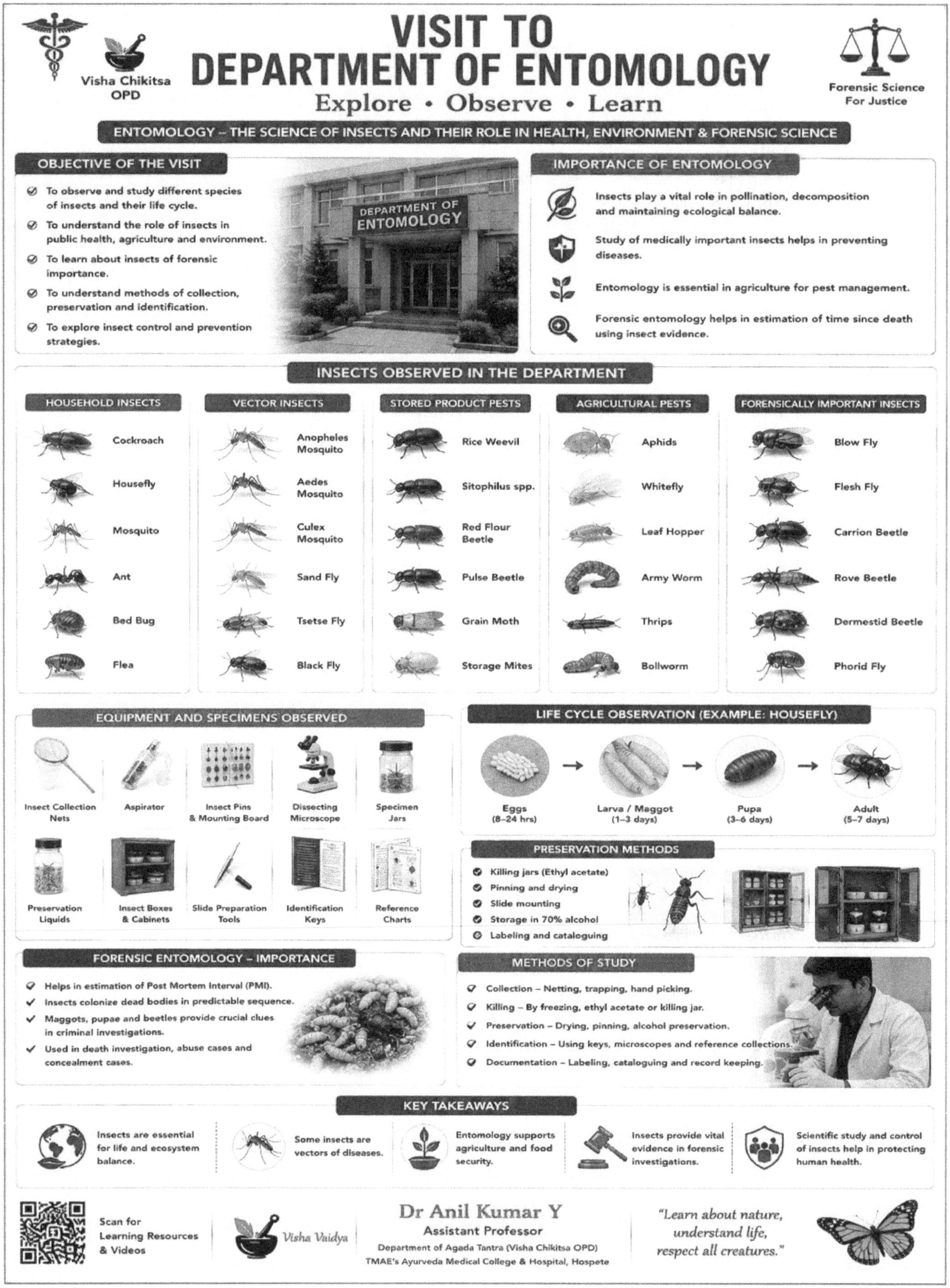
Visha Chikitsa OPD
VISIT TO
DEPARTMENT OF ENTOMOLOGY
Explore • Observe • Learn
Forensic Science For Justice
ENTOMOLOGY – THE SCIENCE OF INSECTS AND THEIR ROLE IN HEALTH, ENVIRONMENT & FORENSIC SCIENCE
OBJECTIVE OF THE VISIT
To observe and study different species of insects and their life cycle.
To understand the role of insects in public health, agriculture and environment.
To learn about insects of forensic importance.
To understand methods of collection, preservation and identification.
To explore insect control and prevention strategies.
DEPARTMENT OF ENTOMOLOGY
IMPORTANCE OF ENTOMOLOGY
Insects play a vital role in pollination, decomposition and maintaining ecological balance.
Study of medically important insects helps in preventing diseases.
Entomology is essential in agriculture for pest management.
Forensic entomology helps in estimation of time since death using insect evidence.
INSECTS OBSERVED IN THE DEPARTMENT
HOUSEHOLD INSECTS
Cockroach
Housefly
Mosquito
Ant
Bed Bug
Flea
VECTOR INSECTS
Anopheles Mosquito
Aedes Mosquito
Culex Mosquito
Sand Fly
Tsetse Fly
Black Fly
STORED PRODUCT PESTS
Rice Weevil
Sitophilus spp.
Red Flour Beetle
Pulse Beetle
Grain Moth
Storage Mites
AGRICULTURAL PESTS
Aphids
Whitefly
Leaf Hopper
Army Worm
Thrips
Bollworm
FORENSICALLY IMPORTANT INSECTS
Blow Fly
Flesh Fly
Carrion Beetle
Rove Beetle
Dermestid Beetle
Phorid Fly
EQUIPMENT AND SPECIMENS OBSERVED
Insect Collection Nets
Aspirator
Insect Pins & Mounting Board
Dissecting Microscope
Specimen Jars
Preservation Liquids
Insect Boxes & Cabinets
Slide Preparation Tools
Identification Keys
Reference Charts
LIFE CYCLE OBSERVATION (EXAMPLE: HOUSEFLY)
Eggs (8–24 hrs)
Larva / Maggot (1–3 days)
Pupa (3–6 days)
Adult (5–7 days)
PRESERVATION METHODS
Killing jars (Ethyl acetate)
Pinning and drying
Slide mounting
Storage in 70% alcohol
Labeling and cataloguing
FORENSIC ENTOMOLOGY – IMPORTANCE
Helps in estimation of Post Mortem Interval (PMI).
Insects colonize dead bodies in predictable sequence.
Maggots, pupae and beetles provide crucial clues in criminal investigations.
Used in death investigation, abuse cases and concealment cases.
METHODS OF STUDY
Collection – Netting, trapping, hand picking.
Killing – By freezing, ethyl acetate or killing jar.
Preservation – Drying, pinning, alcohol preservation.
Identification – Using keys, microscopes and reference collections.
Documentation – Labeling, cataloguing and record keeping.
KEY TAKEAWAYS
Insects are essential for life and ecosystem balance.
Some insects are vectors of diseases.
Entomology supports agriculture and food security.
Insects provide vital evidence in forensic investigations.
Scientific study and control of insects help in protecting human health.
Scan for Learning Resources & Videos
Visha Vaidya
Dr Anil Kumar Y
Assistant Professor
Department of Agada Tantra (Visha Chikitsa OPD)
TMAE's Ayurveda Medical College & Hospital, Hospete
"Learn about nature, understand life, respect all creatures."

PRACTICAL NO. 15

FIELD VISIT REPORT

VISIT TO DEPARTMENT OF ENTOMOLOGY

OBSERVATION OF MEDICALLY IMPORTANT INSECTS AND THEIR PUBLIC HEALTH SIGNIFICANCE

Date of Visit: __________

Place of Visit: ______________________

Name of Institution/Department: ______________________

Faculty Accompanying: ______________________

1. Title of Visit

Visit to Department of Entomology for Observation of Medically Important Insects and Their Public Health Significance.

2. Objectives

1. To understand the scope and importance of Entomology.
2. To observe medically important insects and arthropods.
3. To study insect vectors responsible for disease transmission.
4. To learn methods of vector control and prevention.

3. Introduction

Entomology is the branch of science dealing with the study of insects and arthropods. Medical Entomology focuses on insects that affect human health by causing disease directly or acting as vectors for transmission of infectious diseases.

4. Observations

A. General Information

- Name of Department: ____________________
- Institution: ____________________
- Date of Visit: ____________________
- Guide/Faculty: ____________________

B. Medically Important Insects Observed

Sl. No.	Insect/Arthropod	Disease/Importance
1	Mosquito	Malaria, Dengue, Chikungunya, Filariasis
2	Housefly	Mechanical transmission of diseases
3	Sand Fly	Kala-azar (Leishmaniasis)
4	Flea	Plague
5	Louse	Pediculosis, Typhus
6	Tick	Tick-borne diseases
7	Mite	Scabies
8	Honey Bee	Stings and allergic reactions

C. Specimens and Displays Observed

- Preserved insect collections.
- Life cycle models of mosquitoes.
- Vector identification charts.
- Microscopic specimens.
- Insect breeding and rearing units.
- Educational exhibits on vector control.

D. Life Cycles Observed

Mosquito Life Cycle

1. Egg
2. Larva
3. Pupa
4. Adult

Housefly Life Cycle

1. Egg
2. Larva (Maggot)
3. Pupa
4. Adult Fly

E. Vector Control Methods Observed

Method	Examples
Environmental Control	Removal of stagnant water
Mechanical Control	Mosquito nets, screening
Biological Control	Larvivorous fish
Chemical Control	Insecticides and larvicides
Personal Protection	Repellents and protective clothing

5. Public Health Importance

1. Prevention of vector-borne diseases.
2. Control of disease outbreaks.
3. Environmental sanitation.
4. Community health education.
5. Surveillance of disease vectors.

6. Learning Outcomes

1. Understood the scope of medical entomology.
2. Observed various medically important insects and arthropods.
3. Learned disease transmission by insect vectors.

4. Understood life cycles of important vectors.
5. Appreciated the importance of vector control measures.

7. Conclusion

The visit to the Department of Entomology provided practical exposure to medically important insects, their identification, life cycles, disease transmission and control measures. Entomological knowledge is essential in public health, preventive medicine and toxicology.

8. Result

Observed medically important insects and arthropods, their life cycles, vector-borne diseases and methods of vector control, thereby understanding their significance in public health.

Teacher's Signature

Student's Signature

PRACTICAL NO. 15

FIELD VISIT REPORT

VISIT TO FOLKLORE VAIDYA USING AGADATANTRA CONCEPTS IN VISHA CHIKITSA

Date of Visit: __________

Place of Visit: ______________________

Name of Folklore Vaidya: ______________________

Faculty Accompanying: ______________________

1. Title of Visit

Visit to Folklore Vaidya for Observation of Traditional Visha Chikitsa Practices Based on Agadatantra Principles

2. Objectives

1. To observe traditional methods of Visha Chikitsa practiced by folklore vaidyas.
2. To understand the application of Agadatantra principles in community-based poison management.
3. To study medicinal plants and formulations used in traditional toxicology.
4. To compare traditional knowledge with classical Agadatantra concepts.

3. Introduction

Agadatantra is one of the eight branches of Ayurveda dealing with poisons, poisoning and their management. In many rural areas, folklore vaidyas continue to practice traditional Visha Chikitsa using herbal medicines, local medicinal plants and indigenous knowledge passed through generations. These practices have contributed significantly to community healthcare, especially in the management of snakebite, insect bites and plant poisoning.

4. Observations

A. General Information

- Name of Folklore Vaidya: ______________________
- Place of Practice: ______________________
- Years of Experience: ______________________
- Type of Cases Managed: ______________________

B. Types of Cases Commonly Treated

Sl. No.	Condition	Traditional Management
1	Snake Bite	Herbal formulations and supportive measures
2	Scorpion Sting	Local herbal applications
3	Insect Bite	Plant-based remedies
4	Food Poisoning	Herbal detoxification measures
5	Plant Poisoning	Traditional antidotal preparations

C. Medicinal Plants Observed

Sl. No.	Local Name	Botanical Name	Traditional Use
1	Tulasi	Ocimum sanctum	Supportive treatment
2	Nirgundi	Vitex negundo	Anti-inflammatory use
3	Haridra	Curcuma longa	Wound and poison management
4	Neem	Azadirachta indica	Detoxification support
5	Shirisha	Albizia lebbeck	Described as Visha-hara in Ayurveda

D. Agadatantra Concepts Observed

- Use of Visha-hara (anti-poisonous) herbs.
- Identification of poisonous bites and stings.
- Traditional first-aid measures.
- Use of herbal formulations based on local knowledge.
- Referral of severe cases to hospitals when necessary.

E. Discussion with Folklore Vaidya

Information Obtained

1. Common poisoning cases encountered.
2. Methods of identifying venomous bites.
3. Herbal preparations used in treatment.
4. Source and preparation of medicinal plants.
5. Limitations of traditional treatment.
6. Importance of early referral in severe poisoning cases.

5. Correlation with Agadatantra

Classical Concept	Observation
Visha Lakshanas	Recognition of poisoning symptoms
Visha Hara Dravyas	Use of anti-poisonous herbs
Agada Yogas	Traditional antidotal preparations
Chikitsa Siddhanta	Symptomatic and supportive management

6. Learning Outcomes

1. Understood the role of folklore vaidyas in rural healthcare.
2. Observed traditional Visha Chikitsa practices.
3. Learned about medicinal plants used in poison management.
4. Appreciated the relevance of Agadatantra in community settings.
5. Understood the importance of integrating traditional knowledge with modern medical care.

7. Conclusion

The visit provided valuable exposure to traditional poison management practices and the application of Agadatantra principles in community healthcare. Folklore vaidyas preserve important indigenous knowledge regarding medicinal plants and Visha Chikitsa, while modern medical intervention remains essential in severe poisoning cases.

8. Result

Observed the practices of a Folklore Vaidya in the management of poisoning cases and understood the use of traditional herbal remedies, Agadatantra principles and community-based approaches to Visha Chikitsa.

Teacher's Signature

Student's Signature

PRACTICAL NO. 16

DISCUSSION ON REGIONAL TOXICOLOGICAL, MEDICO-LEGAL AND VISHA CHIKITSA PRACTICES

Date: ____________

Title

Discussion on Regional Preference Topics: Bites and Stings, Substance Abuse, Regional Texts, Regional Visha Chikitsa Practices and Regional Medico-Legal Issues

Aim

To study and discuss region-specific toxicological, medico-legal and Visha Chikitsa practices relevant to the local population.

Objectives

1. To understand common regional poisoning and envenomation cases.
2. To study prevalent substance abuse patterns in the region.
3. To know traditional and regional Visha Chikitsa practices.
4. To understand medico-legal issues commonly encountered in the region.
5. To appreciate regional contributions to Agadatantra knowledge.

Introduction

Regional variations in climate, flora, fauna, occupation, cultural practices and socio-economic conditions influence the pattern of poisoning, bites, stings and medico-legal problems. Understanding these regional issues helps the physician provide appropriate preventive and therapeutic measures.

Observations and Discussion

A. Regional Bites and Stings

Common Cases Observed

Sl. No.	Type	Regional Importance
1	Snake Bite	Common in rural and agricultural areas
2	Scorpion Sting	Frequently seen in dry and semi-arid regions
3	Bee/Wasp Sting	Common during farming and outdoor activities
4	Spider Bite	Occasionally encountered
5	Insect Bites	Common in all regions

Management Principles

- Identification of species when possible.
- First aid measures.
- Early referral to healthcare facilities.
- Administration of Anti-Snake Venom (ASV) where indicated.
- Symptomatic and supportive management.

B. Regional Substance Abuse Patterns

Substance	Commonly Observed Effects
Alcohol	Dependence, liver disease, accidents
Tobacco	Oral cancer, respiratory disorders
Cannabis	Behavioral and psychological effects
Opioids	Dependence and withdrawal symptoms
Inhalants	Neurological complications

Public Health Impact

- Addiction and dependence.
- Domestic and social problems.
- Occupational impairment.
- Increased medico-legal cases.

C. Regional Texts and Traditional Knowledge

Examples

- Local Ayurvedic manuscripts.
- Traditional Visha Chikitsa literature.
- Indigenous medicinal knowledge.
- Folk medicinal practices.

Importance

- Preservation of local healthcare traditions.
- Documentation of medicinal plants.
- Community-based poison management practices.

D. Regional Visha Chikitsa Practices

Common Traditional Practices

- Use of locally available Visha-hara herbs.
- Herbal paste applications.
- Decoctions and internal medications.
- Traditional first-aid methods.
- Community awareness regarding poisonous animals.

Commonly Used Herbs

Herb	Traditional Use
Shirisha	Visha-hara
Haridra	Anti-inflammatory
Tulasi	Supportive treatment
Nirgundi	Local application
Neem	Detoxification support

E. Regional Medico-Legal Issues

Issue	Significance
Snakebite Deaths	Common rural medico-legal problem
Pesticide Poisoning	Agricultural exposure and suicides
Road Traffic Accidents	Frequent medico-legal cases
Alcohol-related Offences	Public health and legal concern
Occupational Hazards	Industry-specific problems
Domestic Violence	Social and legal issue
Food Adulteration	Public health concern

Learning Outcomes

1. Understood region-specific toxicological problems.
2. Learned common bites and stings encountered locally.
3. Studied patterns of substance abuse.
4. Observed traditional Visha Chikitsa practices.
5. Understood important regional medico-legal issues.

Conclusion

Regional knowledge of poisoning, bites, stings, substance abuse and medico-legal issues is essential for effective healthcare delivery. Traditional Visha Chikitsa practices, along with modern medical management, contribute to better community health outcomes.

Result

Studied and discussed regional toxicological, medico-legal and Visha Chikitsa practices, including bites and stings, substance abuse, traditional treatment methods and common medico-legal issues relevant to the region.

Teacher's Signature

Student's Signature

Made easy

Plant Poison

Sl. No.	Poison Category	Common Name	Botanical/Chemical Name	Identification Features	Toxic Principle
1	Plant Poison	Dhattura	Datura metel	Thorny fruit, trumpet-shaped flowers, kidney-shaped seeds	Atropine, Hyoscyamine, Scopolamine
2	Plant Poison	Gunja	Abrus precatorius	Red seeds with black spot	Abrin
3	Plant Poison	Vatsanabha	Aconitum ferox	Conical tuberous root	Aconitine
4	Plant Poison	Karaveera	Nerium oleander	Pink/white flowers, milky latex	Oleandrin
5	Plant Poison	Snuhi	Euphorbia neriifolia	Thick succulent stem, milky latex	Euphorbol esters
6	Plant Poison	Kupilu	Strychnos nux-vomica	Flat circular seeds with silky hairs	Strychnine
7	Plant Poison	Bhallataka	Semecarpus anacardium	Black kidney-shaped fruit	Bhilawanol
8	Plant Poison	Eranda	Ricinus communis	Mottled seeds, spiny capsule	Ricin

Metal & Mineral Poisons

Sl. No.	Poison	Chemical Formula	Identification
1	Arsenic	As_2O_3	White powder, odorless
2	Lead	Pb	Heavy gray metal
3	Mercury	Hg	Silvery liquid metal
4	Copper Sulphate	$CuSO_4$	Blue crystals
5	Zinc Phosphide	Zn_3P_2	Dark gray powder, garlic odor
6	White Phosphorus	P	Waxy yellow substance
7	Red Phosphorus	P	Red powder
8	Aluminium Phosphide	AlP	Gray tablets with garlic odor

Acids

Sl. No.	Acid	Formula	Identification
1	Sulphuric Acid	H_2SO_4	Oily liquid, chars organic matter
2	Nitric Acid	HNO_3	Yellow fumes, yellow stains
3	Hydrochloric Acid	HCl	Colorless liquid, pungent odor
4	Oxalic Acid	$H_2C_2O_4$	Colorless crystals
5	Carbolic Acid	Phenol	Characteristic phenolic odor

Alkalis

Sl. No.	Alkali	Formula	Identification
1	Sodium Hydroxide	$NaOH$	White flakes/pellets
2	Potassium Hydroxide	KOH	White hygroscopic pellets
3	Ammonium Hydroxide	NH_4OH	Strong ammonia smell
4	Calcium Hydroxide	$Ca(OH)_2$	White powder

Hydrocarbons

Sl. No.	Poison	Source	Identification
1	Kerosene	Petroleum product	Characteristic odor
2	Petrol	Petroleum product	Volatile liquid
3	Diesel	Petroleum product	Oily liquid
4	Turpentine Oil	Pine resin	Strong aromatic odor
5	Benzene	Industrial solvent	Sweet aromatic odor

Agrochemicals (Pesticides)

Sl. No.	Poison	Group	Identification
1	Malathion	Organophosphate	Yellow-brown liquid
2	Parathion	Organophosphate	Brown liquid
3	Chlorpyrifos	Organophosphate	Characteristic odor
4	Carbaryl	Carbamate	White powder
5	Carbofuran	Carbamate	Purple granules
6	Endosulfan	Organochlorine	Brown liquid
7	Paraquat	Herbicide	Green liquid
8	Glyphosate	Herbicide	Clear liquid

Household Poisons

Sl. No.	Poison	Common Use	Identification
1	Phenyl	Disinfectant	Characteristic smell
2	Bleaching Powder	Cleaning agent	Chlorine odor
3	Naphthalene Balls	Moth repellent	White balls
4	Toilet Cleaner	Cleaning agent	Strong acidic smell
5	Rat Killer	Rodenticide	Colored granules/cake
6	Mosquito Repellent Liquid	Insecticide	Commercial refill
7	Detergent Powder	Cleaning agent	Foaming powder
8	Camphor	Religious/Household use	White crystalline solid

IMPORTANT MEDICAL LAWS FOR BAMS STUDENTS

1. National Commission for Indian System of Medicine (NCISM) Act, 2020

- Regulates Ayurveda education and practice in India.
- Replaced CCIM (Central Council of Indian Medicine).
- Governs standards of education, ethics, registration, and institutions.

---

2. Drugs and Cosmetics Act, 1940

- Regulates manufacture, sale, and distribution of drugs and cosmetics.
- Includes Ayurvedic, Siddha, and Unani medicines.
- Prevents adulterated and spurious drugs.

---

3. Consumer Protection Act (CPA), 2019

- Protects patients as consumers.
- Medical negligence cases can be filed under CPA.
- Doctors are accountable for deficiency in service.

---

4. Medical Termination of Pregnancy (MTP) Act, 1971 (Amended 2021)

- Governs legal abortion in India.
- Specifies indications, consent, and gestational limits.

---

5. Pre-Conception and Pre-Natal Diagnostic Techniques (PCPNDT) Act, 1994

- Prevents sex selection and female foeticide.
- Regulates ultrasound and prenatal diagnostic procedures.

---

6. Protection of Children from Sexual Offences (POCSO) Act, 2012

- Protects children from sexual offences.
- Mandatory reporting by medical practitioners.

---

7. Mental Healthcare Act (MHCA), 2017

- Protects rights of mentally ill patients.
- Defines procedures for admission, treatment, and consent.

---

8. Transplantation of Human Organs and Tissues Act (THOTA), 1994

- Regulates organ donation and transplantation.
- Prevents commercial organ trade.

---

9. Narcotic Drugs and Psychotropic Substances (NDPS) Act, 1985

- Controls narcotic and psychotropic substances.
- Important in toxicology and medico-legal practice.

---

10. Food Safety and Standards Act (FSSAI), 2006

- Ensures food safety and prevention of adulteration.
- Important for food toxicology practicals.

---

11. Biomedical Waste Management Rules, 2016

- Governs segregation, handling, transport, and disposal of biomedical waste.

---

12. Clinical Establishments Act, 2010

- Regulates registration and standards of hospitals and clinics.

---

13. Registration of Births and Deaths Act, 1969

- Governs issuance of birth and death certificates.

---

14. Human Immunodeficiency Virus (HIV/AIDS) Act, 2017

- Protects confidentiality and rights of HIV patients.

---

15. Indian Evidence Act / Bharatiya Sakshya Adhiniyam (BSA), 2023

- Governs admissibility of medical evidence in court.

---

16. Bharatiya Nagarik Suraksha Sanhita (BNSS), 2023

- Replaced CrPC.
- Important for inquest, medico-legal procedures, dying declaration, etc.

---

17. Bharatiya Nyaya Sanhita (BNS), 2023

- Replaced IPC.
- Includes offences related to hurt, poisoning, negligence, sexual offences, homicide, etc.

---

18. Epidemic Diseases Act, 1897

- Provides powers during epidemic outbreaks.

---

19. Disaster Management Act, 2005

- Important during public health emergencies and disasters.

---

20. Poison Act, 1919

- Regulates possession and sale of poisons.

IMPORTANT SECTIONS OF BNS, BNSS & BSA FOR MEDICAL PRACTICE

I. BHARATIYA NYAYA SANHITA (BNS), 2023

(Replaces IPC)

Section 106 — Causing Death by Negligence

Importance:

- Important section for medical negligence.
- Applies when death occurs due to rash or negligent act.
- Special provision for registered medical practitioners during medical procedures.

Medical Importance:

- Protects doctors from excessive punishment.
- Essential in medico-legal cases and malpractice allegations.

Sections 63–70 — Sexual Offences

Importance:

- Defines rape and related offences.
- Important during examination of sexual assault victims.

Medical Importance:

- Collection of evidence.
- Preparation of medico-legal report.
- Consent and victim examination.

Sections 114–125 — Hurt and Grievous Hurt

Importance:

- Classification of injuries.

Medical Importance:

- Injury certificate preparation.
- Differentiation of simple and grievous injuries.

Sections 85 & 86 — Mental Illness / Unsoundness of Mind

Importance:

- Criminal responsibility in mentally ill persons.

Medical Importance:

- Psychiatric evaluation.
- Medico-legal opinion.

Sections 88–99 — Miscarriage & Foetal Injuries

Importance:

- Offences related to abortion and miscarriage.

Medical Importance:

- Correlation with MTP Act.
- Medico-legal abortion cases.

Section 123 — Poisoning

Importance:

- Administration of poison causing hurt.

Medical Importance:

- Toxicology cases.
- Poison identification and evidence collection.

II. BHARATIYA NAGARIK SURAKSHA SANHITA (BNSS), 2023

(Replaces CrPC)

Section 51 — Medical Examination of Arrested Person

Importance:

- Medical examination permitted only after lawful arrest.

Medical Importance:

- Collection of blood samples.
- Alcohol/drug intoxication cases.
- Preservation of evidence.

Section 52 — Medical Report by Medical Officer

Importance:

- Doctor must submit medico-legal report without delay.

Medical Importance:

- Important in injury, sexual assault, intoxication, and poisoning cases.

Inquest Provisions

Importance:

- Investigation into suspicious or unnatural death.

Medical Importance:

- Postmortem examination.
- Cause of death certification.

Search, Seizure & Documentation Provisions

Importance:

- Digital and video documentation encouraged.

Medical Importance:

- Chain of custody.
- Preservation of forensic evidence.

Arrest and Examination Provisions

Importance:

- Rights of arrested persons.
- Documentation of injuries.

Medical Importance:

- Custodial injury examination.
- Human rights protection.

III. BHARATIYA SAKSHYA ADHINIYAM (BSA), 2023

(Replaces Indian Evidence Act)

Expert Opinion Provisions

Importance:

- Medical practitioners recognized as expert witnesses.

Medical Importance:

- Court testimony.
- Expert medical opinion.

Documentary Evidence

Importance:

- Medical records admissible in court.

Medical Importance:

- OPD/IPD records.
- Certificates.
- MLC reports.
- Postmortem reports.

Electronic Evidence

Importance:

- Digital evidence accepted.

Medical Importance:

- CCTV.
- Electronic prescriptions.
- Digital records.
- Imaging reports.

OVERALL IMPORTANCE TO MEDICAL PRACTICE

Law	Importance to Doctors
BNS	Criminal liability, negligence, injuries, poisoning
BNSS	Investigation, medical examination, MLC procedures
BSA	Evidence, expert witness, medical documentation

Important Note

BNS, BNSS, and BSA came into force from 1 July 2024 replacing IPC, CrPC, and Indian Evidence Act respectively.

ALL THE BEST

"Bridging Classical Ayurvedic Wisdom with Modern Toxicology, Forensic Medicine, and Medico-Legal Sciences for the Physicians of Tomorrow."

आ नो भद्राः क्रतवो यन्तु विश्वतः ।

"May noble thoughts come to us from all directions."
— Ṛgveda 1.89.1

Dr. Anil Kumar Y
B.A.M.S., M.D. (Ayu – Agadatantra)
Assistant Professor, Department of Agadatantra Evam Vidhi Vaidyaka

Visha Vaidya Publications

www.ingramcontent.com/pod-product-compliance
Lightning Source LLC
LaVergne TN
LVHW060031210926
848481LV00013B/3838
* 9 7 9 8 9 0 5 4 0 0 2 1 6 *